I've travelled the world twice over,
Met the famous: saints and sinners,
Poets and artists, kings and queens,
Old stars and hopeful beginners,
I've been where no-one's been before,
Learned secrets from writers and
  cooks
All with one library ticket
To the wonderful world of books.

YOU'RE STILL
A DOCTOR, DOCTOR!

Now retired from his practice and living by the river in Oxfordshire, Dr. Clifford still has light-hearted true tales to tell. There are the holidays at home and abroad, his successful career in broadcasting, colourful portraits of patients and colleagues, and hilarious anecdotes from the past and present.

DR. ROBERT CLIFFORD

◆

YOU'RE STILL A DOCTOR, DOCTOR!

Complete and Unabridged

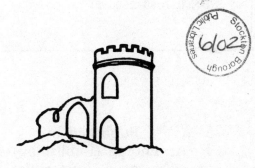

ULVERSCROFT
Leicester

First published in Great Britain in 1989 by
Pelham Books Limited
London

First Large Print Edition
published March 1992
by arrangement with
Pelham Books Limited
London

British Library CIP Data

Clifford, Dr. Robert *1926–*
You're still a doctor, doctor!.—Large print ed.—
Ulverscroft large print series: non-fiction
I. Title
362.1720942

ISBN 0–7089–2600–2

Published by
F. A. Thorpe (Publishing) Ltd.
Anstey, Leicestershire
Set by Words & Graphics Ltd.
Anstey, Leicestershire
Printed and bound in Great Britain by
T. J. Press (Padstow) Ltd., Padstow, Cornwall

*This book is dedicated to the memory
of*
CLIFF PARKER,
*journalist, editor, author, contributor
to many of my books
and steadfast friend for twenty-one
years, a great human being,
much loved by all, sadly missed.*

Prologue

Life is a tragedy, for we are all born eventually to die. We survive our tragedies by laughing at them.

A friend once told me that when he was under the influence of ether he dreamed he was turning over the pages of a great book, in which he knew he would find, on the last page, the meaning of life.

The pages of the book were alternately tragic and comic, and he turned page after page, his excitement growing, not only because he was approaching the answer, but because he couldn't know, until he arrived, on which side of the book the final page would be. At last it came: the universe opened up to him in a hundred words: and they were uproariously funny.

He came back to consciousness crying with laughter, remembering everything. He opened his lips to speak. It was then that the great and comic answer plunged back out of his reach.

Christopher Fry

1

Home Port

IT was a beautiful sunny day on the Thames. We were moored to the bank behind a queue of four boats just above Abingdon Lock. On our right a hire boat flying a German flag was making unsuccessful passes at a post on the opposite side of the river. The post carried a big red notice saying 'DANGER — WEIR'. Perhaps weir means something less hazardous in German.

I was idly gazing along the row of boats in front and saw a tall, bespectacled man step off a boat and disappear over the side. I assumed there must be some new steps down there. Then some inner instinct nagged and I thought I'd better hop off and see what had happened. I walked along the towpath and looked down into the river. There, face downwards with one of his feet on the boat, his head lying over a wooden rail, half in the water, was a man of about seventy.

He was motionless. If he was left where he was he was obviously going to drown — if he wasn't already dead.

I shouted to the lock keeper, who had just started opening the lock gates. He came running, and between us we managed to lift the man up and drag him up the bank. As we laid him down, he opened his eyes, spat out a mouthful of water and said, 'I don't know what happened to me . . . I must have tripped or come over dizzy or something.'

He had a nasty-looking lump under his right eye and I suggested we got an ambulance and sent him to hospital. Although his injury was nothing obviously serious, I thought he might have broken a cheek bone.

Most important, he was alive, which he might well not have been if I had delayed my walk of inspection any longer.

I went back to my boat after seeing the patient safely off in an ambulance. We went through the lock and moored some way on the left-hand bank, downstream of the bridge.

Abingdon is a delightful town, prettier from the river than from the road, with a small theatre in the middle of a group of old buildings, which includes a twelfth-century priory. There are always good moorings on either side of the river, with marvellous facilities on the town bank, including a toilet block that even boasts hot water.

Later that night the Abingdon lock keeper, an old friend of mine, wandered down and came aboard for a nightcap with two of the Dobermann pinschers he bred.

These dogs always frighten me to death, but they were the love of his life and he assured me they wouldn't hurt a fly. Although I could agree that flies might be safe, I wasn't too sure about fat, bald-headed doctors.

'Thanks again, Doc,' he said. 'I don't know what we'd do without you. But how come you always arrive in the nick of time? Better than the Seventh Cavalry, you are.'

By some weird coincidence, whenever I passed through the lock some medical emergency cropped up.

'Look here, Jack,' I said. 'I'm retired now. I don't know whether I'm up to all these medical emergencies.'

'Go on,' said Jack. 'You're still a doctor, Doctor.'

He was right. Although I'd retired to Wallingford six months previously after thirty-three years as a West Country GP, there was no way I could leave medicine completely behind me.

I was on various committees; ex-patients still rang me for advice; at any social functions, as soon as it was known I was a doctor of medicine, symptoms were whipped out more often than handkerchiefs. I was still on a monitoring group of a residential home for the mentally handicapped, I still read the abridged version of the *British Medical Journal* so I wouldn't fall too far behind on medical facts. My favourite page was the obituaries — I used to work out the weekly average of death to try and gauge approximately how many years of retirement I could enjoy.

I resisted all attempts to do locums, life assurance examinations for the DHSS, and other forms of remuneration for doctors who had given up general medical work.

With much heart-searching my wife, Pam, and I left our beloved Tadchester in Somerset where I had been in practice for thirty years and moved to Wallingford in Oxfordshire. There we were fortunate enough to have a house whose garden ran down to the edge of the River Thames, and an old hire boat, the *Sea Grey*, which we had bought to fulfil my ambitions of dividing my time between messing about in boats and writing.

Wallingford, we found, was a delightful place. We'd chosen it after having explored many riverside towns.

You could write a book about the town, in fact, several such books have been written and there are records going back to the ninth century.

It had been a fortified Saxon town in King Alfred's time; William the Conqueror had crossed the river here on his way to London, and his second-in-command had built Wallingford Castle, which survived until Cromwell knocked it down. For many years it was one of the most important castles in the land.

Stephen and Matilda used to fight over it in the twelfth century and on the death of Stephen, Henry (who was King Henry II) became King of England and for a time ruled England from Wallingford Castle.

But that was all in the past.

The present-day attractions are numerous. It is a market town with a Friday market in the square. It has a lovely old town hall and a couple of theatres, one of which spends half its time being a cinema. It also has one of the leading rowing clubs in the country.

There is a wide range of shops, including the headquarters of Habitat and a lovely old family store, five or six absolutely first-class eating places, good river facilities and easy access to London.

Wallingford had so much to offer that there didn't seem to be any reason to go beyond the town boundaries. We bought our clothes in Wallingford, our furniture in Wallingford, we dined in Wallingford, we had our entertainment in Wallingford — theatre and first-class films. It was a real community with a tremendous number of people putting in a great deal of work to provide facilities for their fellow citizens.

The old Regal Cinema had all sorts of functions — badminton, roller skating, and from time to time a flea market. At the Kinecroft Theatre we saw a wonderful rendition of the opera *La Traviata*. The bigger theatre, the Corn Exchange, run by the Sinodian Players, was a delightful playhouse seating about four hundred.

The people who ran the ticket office, the bar staff, the house managers, the lighting experts, were all local people who did it all for nothing.

It was a truly remarkable little town and we counted ourselves lucky to find a house with a river frontage and our own mooring.

2

Maiden Voyage

IT was a great pleasure to be able to walk down to the bottom of the garden to see *Sea Grey* lying at her mooring, a piece of driftwood round one of the front mooring ropes and her fenders bumping against the concrete steps whenever a boat passed.

She looked gleaming white and new. She'd been painted up by the Maid Boat Yard before I'd bought her and, in fact, she was a stately lady of eighteen years and had done her stint as a hire boat.

I had taken her down the river to my friend Andrew Corless at the Sheridan Boat Yard and he'd given her an overhaul and put a pulpit on the foredeck. Not that I'd suddenly gone religious — the pulpit is the front rail of the boat that helps stop you falling off when manoeuvring. He'd also fixed a new back handrail and fixed up navigation lights and a searchlight.

I had been extravagant in adding these lights, and chose the very best quality. They were paid for by a legacy from a wonderful ex-doctor patient, Jackie Dean, who suffered from innumerable complaints and, nursed by her sister, had lived ten years longer than anyone had expected. I wanted to do something special with her gift and the boat navigation lights seemed fitting and proper.

I arranged for my successor in the Tadchester practice, Dr Lichen, to come up from Tadchester and bring up Mary, the sister who had looked after Jackie for so long.

We set off for an evening trip down the river, with supper on board, then came back in the dark with our navigation and searchlights on, travelling peacefully up the river.

I said, 'This is Jackie's present to me, Mary. She's showing us the way home.'

It was a wonderful evening and it felt as if Jackie was with us.

The sky had a peculiar colour that night, and was lit by a great red moon. Mary said this was only the second time in her life that she'd seen such a moon — the day after she saw her first red moon the last Great War had broken out. Happily, there were no new world wars associated with this particular moon.

Cruising along the river in the dark, gliding along slowly so as not to disturb other moored boats, had a special quality of its own. It was almost as if we were travelling in a different world.

On other night trips like this friends would sit on the bow as we headed into the darkness. It was a unique experience with the river wildlife about us. There was something very moving about it.

We were lucky that we lived on part of the Thames that enjoyed the longest stretch between two locks. It was seven miles from Benson Lock, just upriver from Wallingford, down to Cleeve Lock, one of the smallest locks on the Thames.

We could either go upriver, moor below Benson and go into the town, or travel downstream almost to Cleeve Lock, where the Beetle and Wedge Hotel served bar food and had a first-class dining room, and, on the opposite bank, Ye Olde Leather Bottle pub also served excellent food and beer.

We were always made welcome and given a cup of tea at the Sheridan Boat Yard just above the Leather Bottle. We'd known Andrew and his wife Jackie from previous trips over about ten years after they had opened their chandlery and boat yard.

Andrew was much travelled, a bit like Paul Theroux's *Railway Bazaar* but not yet in print. He'd been on the trans-Siberian railway across Japan, down through South America, and across India, but his days of roaming were decreasing as he began producing sons at the rate of knots. To date he'd produced three.

I was lucky to have the Maid Boat Yard, with their big hire fleet, so near to me. They would always cheerfully help me out if I was in trouble and I could take on diesel and water there. Andrew, on whom I looked as my first engineer, took care of overhauls, maintenance, as well as break-downs, new equipment, etc.

Sea Grey was 27 feet long and an Elysian class boat. She was about 9 feet in beam, which meant that she couldn't go up any of the canals as the maximum width of boats for these is 6 feet 8 ins. She had a centre cockpit and wheelhouse, and two things we'd always longed for, a flush toilet (which went into a tank which had to be pumped out) and a shower.

Once the engines had been running for about ten minutes we had hot water in both front and back cabins and in the shower room. The only slight disadvantage to the water set-up was that the pump on any one tap would turn on any other taps which had been left open, including the shower.

When our daughter Jane and some friends were using the boat, one of the boys in her party was very surprised to find it started to rain warm water whilst he was sitting on the toilet in the shower room.

We were to have our maiden voyage with our friends from Devon, Joe and Lyn Church.

What a difference to other boats we'd been on together.

We could push anything we wanted down from the house by wheelbarrow — no more carrying of supplies and equipment for miles.

Our diesel fuel tank held 35 gallons and would last for a couple of weeks' travelling; and our water tank carried 120 gallons, which meant that even with four of us washing and showering we would always have enough for at least a couple of days without having to take on extra water.

It all seemed too good to be true. In the centre cockpit there was a gas refrigerator and in the main back cabin there was a gas fire as well as a gas cooking stove. The boat was extremely well designed and the hot-water tank so well lagged that after a good day's travelling we would still have hot water the following morning.

There were two single berths and a wash basin in the forecabin, then came the shower room and toilet, opposite were some shelves, cupboards and wardrobes. Steps led up to the central cockpit, which was canvas covered and could be opened up. Finally, there was a large rear cabin with two wide bunks, a pull-out table, a sink with hot and cold water, our gas oven and the gas fire.

There was plenty of deck space encompassing the whole boat, providing more than sufficient standing room for the crew manoeuvring the boat through locks.

Having loaded up everything under the sun (including a wine rack in the stern of the boat in the rudder housing) we set off on a beautiful sunny day in June, up through Wallingford to our first stop, Benson Lock, a deep lock with a beautifully maintained garden. Leaving the lock we passed through a lovely stretch of river lined by poplars just after Benson marina and boat house. We moved on, past the Shillingford Bridge Hotel, having first navigated Shillingford Bridge, to enter a stretch of river that wound through trees and meadows, passing what had once been a very stately home on the starboard side, now divided into three houses.

Further up the river we passed the entrance to the river Thames, and our next lock was Days Lock, where the lock keeper, Taffy, and his attractive ginger-haired wife always gave us a great welcome.

Taffy was a great RNLI stalwart. Apart

from several fund-raising functions he had organised from his own lock, we had come across him raising money at Henley and various other spots in the year. Each year he would collect something in the order of £25,000 for the lifeboat fund.

He was also nationally famous for his 'Pooh' stick races from the footbridge just below the lock.

We moored for our first night about half way between Days Lock and Clifton Hampden Lock. There was a lovely stretch of water meadow opposite a Cheshire Home.

It was a delightful place for dogs. Joe and Lyn had brought their border terrier and we'd brought Bertie, our white haired terrier and they were having the time of their lives. There were some lovely little beaches, rat- and rabbit-holes, as well as the river: it was a dog's paradise.

We were so far away from habitation that we were rarely bothered by fishermen or walkers. It was at least two miles to Clifton Hampden bridge and the Barley Mow made famous by Jerome K. Jerome's *Three Men in a Boat*.

We had an early morning breakfast, then travelled up river through Clifton Hampden Lock to the deep lock at Culham, with a glimpse of some beautiful barns and the multi-pastel-shaded Culham House. A slow cruise through the lock cut ended on a broad sweep of river leading into Abingdon.

Approaching Abingdon by river is quite beautiful. You first come to some of the oldest parts of Abingdon, with almshouses, churches and various other old buildings lining the river bank. There's one of the best chandleries on the river below the bridge, then on past the bridge on the left bank there's a park and a swimming pool and mooring for a good mile on the right.

We paid for a night's mooring in Abingdon, and this included a free ticket to Abingdon jail. (This didn't mean we were incarcerated for the night — the jail's been converted to a sports centre!)

Many a time previously we'd lunched at the Nag's Head pub on Abingdon Bridge, shopped in town, then gone above Abingdon Lock to moor for the night where there are open fields, streams and waterfalls.

Sadly for us, but due to promotion for him, our old friend the keeper at Abingdon Lock, Jack, had gone down river to run the old Windsor Lock. As a general principle the further you went down the river the larger it became, and the locks were much busier. We tended to go up-stream where it was less crowded and the scenery more rural.

One problem I had to contend with on this maiden voyage was that once again I had a kidney stone, and, hoping to pass it, I was drinking gallons of water.

All this water meant that I had to get up in the night from time to time, and rather than disturb Joe and Lyn, who were in the forecabin, next to the toilet, I used to loosen the side covers in the cockpit and (albeit against the rules) would try and increase the volume of the river Thames. My symptoms told me I was near to passing the stone, so I stepped up my drinking rate.

One night I crept out at about two in the morning, undid the hatch covers, took up the appropriate posture and started to discharge my cargo into the Thames. Suddenly there was a tremendous splash as a rock plunged into the river, accompanied by a hoot of laughter.

'Your stone's gone all right now, Skipper,' said Joe from the bunk cabin.

Apparently he'd been sitting up half the night waiting for me to lean over the side. Once I was literally in full stream he had thrown in a boulder to encourage me.

In fact, I did not pass this particular stone until several weeks later.

Fortunately, apart from the first two stones that I had (one of which I passed in the middle of the Sahara and was absolute agony), further stones never seemed to bother me much. They caused only discomfort rather than pain.

Above Abingdon Lock we passed Nuneham Courteney, a beautiful old building with a folly and acres of landscaped fields. Radley College boathouse soon appeared, then we tackled the biggest lock on the river, Sandford Lock. A short cruise took us on to Iffley Lock, one of the prettiest locks which still had rollers to push the skips and punts over by hand, then we chugged down through Oxford, under Folly Bridge and into the town itself. The river here was almost like a street, with houses and allotments on each bank. We motored up to Osney Lock, which is followed by Osney Bridge, the lowest bridge on the river and which must have nearly decapitated many boaters. One year, on a hire boat, when Jane was about four years old, we had forgotten she was on the top deck, only remembering when we were halfway under the bridge. Fortunately she had the good sense to lie flat. We could have had a catastrophe.

We continued along the river cut up to Bossoms Boat Yard, where the river widened with the vast area of Port Meadows on the right bank which looked like the Camargue with horses and cows — it was a different world. We passed the Perch Inn on our left, which could be reached by an old landing stage, and journeyed on up to Godstow Lock, the last of the automatic locks. The lock keeper here is a fellow author and has written a first-class book on the middle Thames.

Through Godstow Lock, we passed the ruined priory, a difficult bridge, then the famous Trout Inn where you could get smoked-salmon sandwiches and where everybody who was anybody went to see and be seen. Starlets, dons, actors, politicians, all the fashionable, would sit round in the grounds with its tumbling waterfalls, peacocks and giant trout.

Leaving Godstow Lock we joined a completely different kind of Thames. It wound and twisted and from then on all the locks were manually operated and everything seemed to be at a slower pace. When the lock keepers were at lunch or were out working on the sluices we worked the locks ourselves.

The river steadily narrowed and on this first voyage we were blessed all the time by sunshine. We passed on, winding our way through countryside with marvellous views. From Kings Lock, the first of the manual locks, we journeyed to Eynsham. Our next lock was Pink Hill Lock having first passed a great reservoir on the left bank. Further on up river was a huge caravan/mobile home park on the right bank stretching upstream and ending at the Ferry Boat Inn. This view was unsightly, and not in keeping with this gentler part of the Thames. It was like a sudden lump of suburbia smack in the middle of the countryside. However, this was balanced by the amount of pleasure it must have given to the hundreds of people who came to stay there. It was ideal for family holidays.

A boat such as *Sea Grey* called for a certain amount of daily maintenance. I know nothing about engines and am no good at anything mechanical and had to be instructed on all the various things I had to do.

Each day I had to tighten two screws to make sure there was plenty of grease on the propeller shaft. I had to check the water level in the exchange radiator tank, and the oil level. I had to check the filter where the water-cooling system brought water in from the river, and clean it of any leaves or debris that might be choking it.

I had to start up the bilge pump to see if any bilge water came out from the bilge. The engine compartment was shut off from the rest of the boat and was not connected to the bilge area. If you pumped out your engine compartment in the same way you would have polluted the river with oil, so it had to be done on to the bank into some receptacle where it could be disposed of.

Normally there was nothing of any quantity in the engine compartment, just a little oily water in the channel at the bottom.

On our third day out, however, I noticed that we had collected a pool of blue fluid, not in the bottom of the engine compartment, but in an isolated area on one side. I thought it strange it didn't drain away and eventually I tackled the offending liquid with a mug and bucket. I managed to clear out several buckets and chucked the contents on to the bank, only to have the space fill up again. It also seemed to have a peculiar smell.

Joe, who knows much more about things mechanical than I do, was holding himself with laughter. 'Do you realise what's happened, Skip?' he said.

'No,' I replied.

'I'm afraid our flush toilet mustn't be

flushed any more,' he chuckled. 'The holding tank is leaking into the engine compartment.'

And so it was. So, for the rest of our voyage, having liberally filled the engine compartment with Dettol, we had to go back to using public toilets, banks and bushes and when we got back home the Maid Boat Yard fitted a new bottom to our effluent tank.

Otherwise this first trip on our new boat was absolute heaven. The river was almost empty. We cruised up to Newbridge, having a meal at the Rose Revived on my birthday, past Radcott, where there'd been a terrible battle during the Civil War (you could almost feel and see Cavaliers and Roundheads fighting on the bridge). Then as far as we could go with our boat, the last lock, St John's Lock, and on to Lechlade town, whose church stood out for miles.

Joe, who wasn't satisfied that we'd gone far enough, hired a rowing boat for the day and rowed it up to Cricklade.

We had a couple of days at Lechlade then ambled slowly down river, mooring each night out in the wild, enjoying pub lunches en route, eating on the boat at night to classical music on our tape recorder with lovely sunsets and unbroken beautiful weather.

Finally, we drifted back to our home territory, Abingdon, Culham, Clifton Hampden, Days, Benson Lock and Wallingford Bridge, easing up as we passed the Maid Boat Yard. Slowly we nudged our way (with perfect manoeuvring by the skipper) to our own landing stage at the bottom of the garden.

How very, very lucky we were. The sun doesn't always shine but it had for us those ten days and it had been quite perfect.

3

Taking It Easy

AMONG the greatest joys of retirement are not having to get up early in the morning, not having to work weekends and, above all, not being called out of bed at night.

It took me some weeks to adjust to the fact that my sleep was not going to be disturbed. I felt guilty about enjoying this luxury after so many years of broken nights.

I love the mornings. Our radio alarm is set for 8 o'clock but the central heating gently coming on at 7 a.m. usually wakes me. About the same time I hear the thud of the morning papers falling from the letter box, accompanied by a growl from Bertie, our West Highland terrier. Confined to the kitchen at night, Bertie cannot make his usual terrifying leap at the letterbox, but his growl shows that the guardian of the house is up and alert

25

and ready to take on all comers.

About 7.30 a.m. I hear the postman lean his bike against the wall then a patter as he pushes the day's post through the door. I try and guess how many letters have been delivered, hoping for a win on the football pools or at least a £50 premium bond prize.

Usually it is bills and a fistful of circulars which begin: 'You have been specially selected to take part in a draw for an enormous amount of money providing you take on approval a priceless book (or some other exclusive and valuable item) for half its worth.' A tremendous number of people want to insure me, give me unsecured loans or invest my money for me. With the wood pulp involved in the production of the circulars, it is a wonder there are any trees left standing.

I am spared the mass of giveaway medical magazines that used to fill my dustbin when I was in practice. Now I have some time on my hands I would quite enjoy them. But on asking why these journals were no longer arriving, I was informed that now I was retired I would have to pay for them.

I still receive the *British Medical Journal*, but this is the retired version and does not include the jobs section, which was the only thing I used to read.

I am no longer interested in such papers as 'Cytopathogenic Protein in Filtrates for Cultures of Propionibacterium' or 'Acnes Isolated from Patients with Kawasaki Disease', though, to be honest, even when I was at my medical and intellectual peak I wouldn't have understood them.

The radio alarm goes off at 8 o'clock to be followed by the news headlines, and this is the signal for my wife, Pam, to get up and make me a cup of tea. This sounds like male chauvinism at its worst, but it is by mutual agreement.

A patient once gave me a teasmade and I loved the early-morning drama of it. You were first awakened as it started to bubble. The bubbling increased in tempo until the final climax of water coming to the boil, steam gushing out and the kettle tipping into the pot. At the same time a light came on and the alarm rang. It was just like a small volcano going off in your ear. It must have been invented by someone who lived near the San Andreas

Fault who, knowing that one day they were going to be in a real earthquake, could practice by having a small one every morning.

I loved the teasmade, but Pam hated it. Not only did she lie awake all night listening for it, almost jump out of her skin when the alarm, light and teamaking all suddenly burst into action, but also had to suffer a rotten cup of tea because the pot hadn't been warmed first. She much prefers to get up and make a good cup of tea herself.

On the rare occasions that I actually get up with a fit of conscience and make the tea, it seems to unsettle her for the day, so I lie back and enjoy being spoilt.

While Pam is brewing up, Bertie is let out into the garden for morning ablutions. Then, as Pam enters the bedroom with the morning post, papers and tea, he comes hurtling on to the bed, has a quick lick of my nose then dashes off to look out of the window, front paws on the sill, back legs up straight, like a pair of white jodhpurs.

From the window, Bertie has a

panoramic view of all the ground down to the river. We have a lawn in front of the house, then the service road for our row of houses. Beyond this is a long lawn leading to some concrete hardstanding, a further stretch of lawn, a public right of way and finally a grassy bank and the concrete steps of our mooring with a small slipway where our boat, *Sea Grey*, rocks gently at her moorings.

The right of way is a favourite walking place for dogs, and Bertie, from the security of the bedroom, can threaten any canine. From behind the window, he doesn't care how big they are.

People do not always appreciate that the right of way is through someone's garden so dogs tend to be slipped off leads as soon as they leave the main boat yard, one garden away, rather than kept restrained for another hundred yards until they reach the fields and towpath proper.

It does mean that we have some of the best manured grass in the district and it's important to inspect your shoes carefully if you walk down to the river.

Picnickers and fishermen do not always

quite appreciate that I haven't actually cut and trimmed my lawn just for them, and that there are several miles of other river bank at their disposal. One of my neighbours tried the tactful approach and asked a very persistent group of picnickers if it would be all right if he took his tea round to their house!

The vast majority of people are careful, but the small minority seem hell bent on destruction and will uproot anything uprootable and pinch anything movable.

Now and again I protest if I find a dozen bikes on my bank with their owners scrabbling all over my boat. My remonstrations are usually followed by a posse of small boy cyclists, riding up and down the road shouting 'Fatty!' or 'Baldy!' every time they pass the house. It's very annoying when you're both fat and bald.

Any of them who ask permission to fish are given it and we rarely move anyone on if they are harmlessly enjoying themselves. We feel very privileged to enjoy the facilities we have and it seems a pity not to share them.

Our concrete hardstanding is a legacy

from the last war. It runs right from the boatyard and on through the front lawns-cum-water-meadows of the last six houses of the cul-de-sac. American troops had used it to practise river crossings and bridge building.

Our neighbour, a retired physician, asked a builder for an estimate to remove his bit. The builder quoted £50 and said he would have it done the next afternoon. Three days later they were still hard at it with power drills and bulldozers — the concrete was 12 feet thick.

Back to bed. I read the post and newspaper headlines then Pam appears again with my breakfast; cereal and a piece of toast with honey. She really spoils me, but it does mean that breakfast is now out of the way.

A friend, Trevor Robinson, once staying with us, watched this ritual and then said 'My God, Bob, you're lucky to have her.' I replied 'She's lucky to have me.' 'Yes,' said Trevor, 'but you're luckier than she is.'

By the time I've bathed, washed, shaved and dressed, it's almost coffee time. After that, there's the rest of the day to play with.

Pam takes Bertie for his daily walk along the towpath. I square my conscience by saying it's good for her hip — she had a hip replacement some years ago.

On his walk, Bertie meets some of the dogs he's uttered abuse at earlier in the morning. He has an infallible technique if he meets a really big dog — he jumps straight in the river and hides under the bank.

One day we lost him completely and he was found by a lady who kept a horse by the towpath, shivering in the water almost hidden from view.

But all people and most dogs are Bertie's friends and he races up and down with Lally, Bock and Lilly, his three special friends, full of the joys of doghood.

Meanwhile I check the boat's moorings, pump out the bilge if necessary and generally mess about.

About once a week we have lunch at the delightful Traps winebar in Wallingford, a place to meet friends as well as to eat and drink. It is underneath the Lamb Arcade, an old hotel rescued by the community and developed into a collection of about twenty antique and craft shops, with a first-class secondhand bookshop and a restaurant on the top floor.

Near the Lamb is the lovely old coaching inn, The George, which way back in about 1200 was owned by a Mr Baynton. Pam's maiden name was Baynton and we always hoped that one day, through some ancestral link, we would find we owned it.

There are many first-class eating places in Wallingford. Stoney's down by the bridge compares with any London restaurant. Across the road behind Wallingford Bridge, Boats is the curry house. There are also first-class Indian, Chinese and Greek restaurants. Many of the pubs serve full meals and bar food. There is Upstairs Downstairs in the precinct and the Egon Ronay guide *Have a Bite* recommended Annie's Restaurant, in the Wantage Road.

The old Row Barge pub changed its name to the Little House and produced a full-blown dining room. In addition there are several cafés, sandwich and pie shops.

Eating must appear high on the list of any industries in Wallingford.

Market day is Friday with stalls piled with fruit, veg and flowers; there's also a fish stall and the usual accompanying array of clothes, cooking utensils and other nicknacks for sale.

We have our own excellent fresh fish and game shop coupled with a delicatessen shop, and half a dozen butchers some of whom still wear traditional boaters.

I started both a Philosophy class and an English class but, through various other commitments, reluctantly had to give them up. I particularly missed the English class which consisted of twenty-eight ladies and me — just the right proportion.

Wallingford is famous for its authors. Rex Warner, who wrote *Aerodrome*, was still alive when I arrived in the town, but unfortunately I never met him. Agatha Christie's boathouse is a hundred yards from our garden, and Jerome K. Jerome lived across the river in Ewelme. I hoped that some of this writing aura might rub off on me.

Wallingford Castle, or what is left of it, has been opened up as a park and you can stroll round the grounds climbing to the highest point after crossing the drawbridge, leading to a platform where there is a panoramic view for miles around.

Fundamentally, I am lazy and I find that Wallingford has all the facilities for busily doing nothing, at which I claim to be an expert.

Our Norman first came into our lives in Tadchester, when I was laid off work with chest pains, just before I had a coronary bypass. I was unable to do any heavy physical work and we needed some help in the garden. Norman volunteered and gradually became part of the family. His duties eventually included staying in the house and looking after Bertie (who loved him) when we were away.

After many years of working as a printer, he could have retired comfortably on his pensions but he preferred to do two or three days' work a week, as well as maintaining a big allotment, so that he could travel to the four corners of the earth which he literally did. This year he is off to Barcelona in the spring, Moscow and Leningrad in the autumn, squeezing in his annual month's touring in France in between.

To our great delight he had moved to Wallingford before us, since two of his children lived nearby. When we arrived he immediately resumed all his former tasks. He'd sometimes come round for a meal or we'd dine out together. We had a lovely couple of days on the river, just the three of us in *Sea Grey*, pottering up to Sandford Lock, just below Oxford.

He was the first of the clan of old friends and relatives who started to settle around us in Wallingford.

By sheer chance an old friend, Joan Gore, who we'd known since before the War, arrived in Wallingford. She didn't come because she knew us, in fact I don't think she knew we were there. She was later followed by her brother and sister. Then one of those strange coincidences, if they are coincidences, happened. I had some cousins up north — three boys. I hadn't seen them since my Bevin Boy days back in 1945 – 46, when they were tiny short-trousered tearaways. One of them, the oldest, Anthony, took a degree at Manchester University, then went into the air force as a pilot where, amongst other things, he won the Nato bombing award.

After doing a spell in the RAF he was seconded to the Saudi Air Force and he and his wife, Eunice, stayed out in Saudi for another ten years.

They had two sons just leaving school in the Isle of Man and felt if a job turned up on their next leave, they'd have to stay. If they left it much later the settling down in England again would be even more difficult and although they loved the Saudi life, they appreciated they couldn't stay there for ever. One day I had a 'phone call from Anthony's father to say Anthony had moved to Wallingford, 300 yards away from us — it was quite incredible.

They turned out to be a delightful couple, and it was a great comfort to know we had blood relatives in the town. Anthony was employed by a merchant bank and Eunice was working for the British Trust for Conservation

Volunteers, which continues to grow in importance and makes a tremendous contribution to present-day society.

I wonder, are these things coincidences? A lot of philosophers have believed in the existence of overall patterns to our lives and that some people will keep turning up in them. Certainly I have noticed that there are some people I am always bumping into. And what, for example, are the chances of two cousins who hadn't met for nearly forty years, arriving unplanned in the same town to live 300 yards from each other?

Tony Murphy, a friend with whom I was at medical school, is one such example. When I was in practice in Tadchester, we twice bumped into him when we were on holiday in St Ives and he was on leave from his work in Mombassa. He, like Anthony and Eunice, felt that you had to return home at some stage and, by chance, he came to a practice in Reading and Pam bumped into him one day in a supermarket.

So we really were blessed and felt we did belong, in addition we had excellent neighbours and the whole small cul-de-sac we lived in, looked out for each other. We were indeed very lucky.

It all added to the fullness of life. It meant at the least that when one or all of us had flu, we could make sympathetic noises down the phone to each other. We weren't isolated strangers in a foreign land.

But Wallingford was that sort of place. It had an aura of something special about it, quite what I don't know, but I know of no other place where there are so many community projects going on and with so many people giving up their time voluntarily to see that they are carried out.

I remember so well the words of three wise old men many years before when asked for the answer to life's problems or society's problems. They said: 'It's not better systems, it's just better people we need,' and Wallingford certainly seemed to have more than its share of these.

I have always maintained that cheaper travel and easier access to different countries could be a main factor in achieving world peace. We would find that people who lived in other countries weren't strange or alien creatures, but ordinary people like you and me.

The twinning of towns was a great step in that direction. Luxeil les Bains was twinned with Wallingford and when their orchestra came over to play in the town, we put up a couple of the visiting musicians. Our guests were a delightful girl from Reims, who was studying the cello, and a professor from Montpelier, who had the most superb baritone voice.

We made two new friends and there were two new places on the Continent where we would always be welcome; and they, of course, knew that they would always be welcome to return here.

They gave us a splendid concert in the Corn Exchange, a theatre-cum-cinema, despite a horrendous forty-hour coach journey.

Perhaps we'd return the visit when Wallingford visited Luxeil les Bains.

I did learn one thing from their stay: I'd always pronounced Reims like 'reams', but the French pronunciation is 'rance' — why, I don't know. This reminded me of the day I tried to find the Devon village of Woolfardisworthy — nobody knew it when I asked for it by name, apparently locally it was always pronounced as Woolsery.

By comparison Rance for Reims is just small beer. French beer, of course.

4

Family Affairs

IT was our turn to be hosts at Christmas. I really am turning into an old stick-in-the-mud.

The children with their new homes had bagged the last two Christmases. We had the first with daughter Jane and son Trevor at Brighton, where they completely spoiled us. The only disadvantage about their accommodation is that it's up four flights of stairs, which would have been fine if we hadn't had Bertie with us — it's an awful long way to go to take him to find a lamp-post and a much longer way to find a precious piece of greensward to complete his daily rituals.

They were very proud of their flat and really gave us a smashing time.

The next year it had to be the turn of our other son, Paul, and his wife, Gill.

Their home is at Cirencester, where we had a repeat of the same formula. We were extremely lucky that we were able to gather as a family on these occasions. Daisy May, our new granddaughter was, of course, the centre of attention this Christmas, but being only about five months old, she wasn't too aware of what was going on.

So now it was our turn. They were all coming, Jane, Trevor, Gill, Paul, Daisy May, and Gill's parents, Eddie and Liz. We put mattresses from the boat in my study for Paul and Gill, Trevor slept on a camp bed in the lounge and Jane shared a room with Daisy May and it was her Christmas. Her main present was a Noddy Car — I think we were all more excited about it than she was.

Gill was ready with her ciné camera to film Daisy May getting up on Christmas morning and finding the car. Through the lens, Gill was able to capture for ever the look of astonishment on Daisy May's face at seeing this new gift, of her exploring it and climbing into it.

We had a great Christmas and we were

so lucky that our children — of course, they were no longer children — were getting on so well.

Trevor had turned into a fine actor. I thought his series *Star Cops* on BBC 2 was excellent. It was hoped that it would go on to BBC 1 and they would do a second series — perhaps it will, but nothing to date.

He made a film called *Drowning by Numbers*, which he said his mother wouldn't want to see as his wife drowns him at sea. In fact, when they were filming it off Southwold on the Suffolk coast in October they hadn't rehearsed the drowning scene explicitly before they did the take and it was very realistic — he accidentally took a mouthful of water the first time she pushed him under and he really thought he was going to drown. Then, in the cold of October, he had to lie naked on the beach while they filmed him being resuscitated, or filmed people trying to resuscitate him because in the story he perishes.

(Not in the script, his wife, who had done this dastardly deed, nearly died of hypothermia.)

He was enjoying a variety of engagements: an advertisement for Schweppes in New Zealand; an educational film for the Inland Revenue; a commercial for a washing machine where he was in drag as one of two ugly sisters; a commercial in Dublin; and something he could really get his teeth into — three months at the Manchester Royal Exchange Theatre in *Twelfth Night*, where he was to play Sir Toby Belch.

Paul had taken a new job, when an opportunity came up. This was a step forward for him and just his cup of tea. He joined a newish firm selling an American product — and it meant Paul going off to Chicago two or three weeks a year for training, and a business conference in Florida. The firm was going to go into Europe and he was already destined to accompany one of the senior officials from the firm to visit Austria, Switzerland, Italy and Spain.

It seemed an extremely good company and when Paul was making his first trip to Chicago, they arranged for Paul and Gill to stay the night at a Manchester hotel so Gill could see him off.

Paul loved Chicago, and what I thought was most refreshing was that the American head of the firm talked to him and explained that they were a firm that held on to the old values; they weren't 'fly by night' sales people; they had a product they believed in. He said 'For example, we've just asked our suppliers to increase their prices, which sounds crazy, but it isn't. They give us a good product and we don't want them to go out of business. We want the best, and so when one of my workmen comes in and complains that the materials he's working with aren't good enough, I'm not upset by this, I'm pleased. It means he believes in what he's doing, and I see he gets the better stuff, and that's the way we work.' This is similar to my own philosophy and I know it tallies with Paul's; I wouldn't wish him any other job. It's quite amazing that in a three-year period he's moved from a dull, routine job, from which he seemed to have no escape, to a post with an electronic component firm, slowly building up his confidence and travelling all over England, to now, a couple of years later, an international company salesman, travelling all over the world.

At the same time Gill, a trained jeweller and artist, had begun to sell card designs to Gordon Fraser. They, too, seemed extremely nice people to work for and she made enough from her first batch of cards to buy herself a little car. This meant she would be able to come and see us more often and, now her husband was a world traveller, she would have a bit more freedom of movement.

Jane was still the night stage doorkeeper at the Brighton Theatre Royal and although Jane always did find kind things to say about people, she met many famous theatrical people on pre-London runs down there and she always spoke of how nice they were to her.

During the day she plugged away at her dressmaking business, cutting out and designing clothes, then taking to market.

It was extremely heavy going and working on her own wasn't too much fun. Although she had some very good days, by the time she'd earned a bit of money, she had usually run out of material, so most of her takings went into purchasing material for her next batch. Her profit margins were too small and she wasn't a businesswoman.

She'd become a very able seamstress but was beginning to show signs of wanting to travel and this costs money. She was nursing a great ambition to go to New Zealand and although I had tentatively brought the subject up in the past, this time she accepted my advice and went on a shorthand-typing and word-processing course. This would mean that wherever she went she could always do some temping. It wouldn't stop her carrying on with her dressmaking once she'd learnt her new found skills, but at least she'd have another string to her bow.

In the Easter holidays, she had a marvellous week skiing in Austria with her friend, also called Jane. Prior to her holiday she was almost a vegetarian, and was not very good at getting up in the mornings, but a week in Austria made all the difference. They were up at 7 a.m. to tackle steeper and steeper slopes, and they came home in the evenings literally exhausted. Most of the food on offer was meat, potatoes and dumplings, and for that week all thoughts of being a vegetarian vanished. Both girls ate every bit.

They had only one accident, when they came down one of the steepest slopes at about 100 miles an hour and ran into each other, but apart from a few bruises they were both all right.

Of the fourteen group members that started the course only six survived. On the last day the instructor took them up a very high mountain (from Jane's description you'd have thought it was Everest). He just said, 'Right ho, off you go,' and off they went. But they came back sunburnt, full of beans and raring to go.

Pam integrated well into Wallingford. We both joined the Sinodian Players as non-active players — this was the nearby theatre-cum-cinema run by local people. Pam also helps out at the local Oxfam shop and the Wallingford Museum, which puts on two or three excellent exhibitions a year. They were held in one of the oldest houses in the town, the Old Flint House.

I have become, I'm afraid, very lazy. I'm not a great gardener, but will cut the grass when necessary. I was very happy fiddling about with the boat and have helped out with the annual regatta. The first two regattas in which we were involved, although held on the first weekend in May, were bitterly cold.

We were the 'long start', which meant I had to take *Sea Grey* to pick up various items of equipment — tents, chairs, etc. — and people who were running the start, and take them down river to the point where the long river races used to be started, opposite Carmell College, a boys' boarding school.

I never realised what a complicated business it was.

There were about six or seven radio links with various points down the river, and teams of Sea Scouts had to man the stake boats, from which they held on to the back of race boats and steadied them before they set off.

I had some help from Bernard and Joyce Walter, some old friends from Woolhampton. Bernard helped row the boys to and from the stake boats, and our boat, being the only warm place to shelter, became a mobile canteen. Joyce made over a hundred cups of tea for these little lads, who came on board with chattering teeth and gradually warmed up before they had to return to do their next stint on the boats.

The third year we were due to be at the long start with the biggest entry Wallingford had ever had for its regatta — 250 boats. I think it was about the third largest in the country and there were going to be races from eight in the morning till seven o'clock at night.

We had good cooking facilities on *Sea Grey* and anticipating warming up little boys and starting officials in bitterly cold weather, Pam got in a whole pile of beefburgers, with Coke for the younger members and whisky for the starters and senior officials. We set off, leaving our mooring at seven o'clock in the morning, and went down river as far as the Spastic Training College, which was the finishing post where all the officials and equipment were waiting. We picked up all the necessary gear and officials and headed back up river, ready for the first race at eight o'clock.

We had jumpers, anoraks, mackintoshes — everything for cold, wet weather — and it turned out to be one of the sunniest, hottest days of the year. It was absolutely glorious.

Fortunately the fridge was working and by chance we had a dozen cans of beer on board. I don't know how many races actually took place but with 250 crews and quarter finals, semi-finals and finals, the regatta seemed endless. What impressed me most were all the people who gave their time to this exhausting day. By the time all the races were over and we had collected up the equipment, plus one odd rowing boat we found abandoned on the way, it was about 8.30 pm. when we got back to the race finish at the Spastic headquarters, a lovely building with a beautiful lawn, loaned by the Society for many of the bigger social occasions held in Wallingford.

We got back to our mooring at about nine.

People were still working, pulling up buoys, taking down flags and markers — for many it had been approximately a fourteen-hour day, a real community effort.

Luckily this year, all had gone well. The previous year I'd commented on how refreshing it was to see all these young men tugging their hearts out against each other, literally hundreds of them, and what a good omen it was for the future etc., not knowing that at that very moment officials were shutting the bar at race headquarters because some louts had started to throw things about and abuse the people who were serving. There was a fight with the police, arrests and all sorts of goings on.

On the day of this regatta such problems had been forestalled. Some 'heavies' had been brought in to protect the establishment so there were no troubles at base and a most successful day was had by everyone.

I contributed very little, just appearing for a day with my boat, enjoying an outing in the sunshine.

Wallingford is certainly not short of community spirited people who give a tremendous amount of time to organise and set up this occasion. Because of people like this we are able to enjoy the theatres, the carnival, music in Wallingford Castle and St Peter's Church and many other functions.

So long as communities like this flourish I think society has nothing to fear. If there were more places with the spirit and enterprise of Wallingford, how much less the troubles in society would be.

5

Encore Portugal

WE felt that we would like some sun on our backs before the year closed. Having enjoyed one winter holiday in Portugal, we thought we'd go for another at the tag end of the season, so we set off for Lagos on the Algarve.

We'd loved the previous holiday in Faro, the capital of the Algarve, in the winter. We realised we were rather spoilt then as there weren't too many planes about and the planes weren't too big. On this particular trip we were on a wide-bodied jet and it seemed to arrive at Faro airport with about six other wide-bodied jets, all unloading at the same time and there was a tremendous scramble for luggage. You have to be fit to travel by plane nowadays.

There were scores of buses waiting to take passengers to their hotels.

YSDD5

Our departure from Faro airport at the end of our holiday was worse than our arrival as all the communication systems, the computer boards detailing flight times, had broken down, a couple of planes had engine trouble and the passengers had been waiting twelve hours to board.

There was a seething mass of people all wondering if they were going to fly out that night, and whoever was speaking over the public address system would never win a prize for English pronunciation: it was unintelligible.

We had a two-hour journey to our hotel, dropping people off at various places en route, passing near Albufeira which now, alas, could be mistaken for a popular Spanish resort with thousands of hotels and thousands more going up. We caught a beautiful view of the fishing town of Portimao with a huge sardine restaurant at the side of the bridge. There were rows and rows of tables and a hazy sardine smoke floating above the whole area — it looked most appetising. We had to drop some people off at Praia da Rocha which, although having lovely hotels and beautiful beaches, seemed like Albufeira trying to catch up with Spain.

And then on to our hotel, the Hotel de Lagos, which was quite beautiful and seemed to have twice as many lounges, all beautifully clean and appointed, as it did residents.

Our room was pleasant, but the dining room was rather disappointing. It was a bit like being back at school: you had to queue for a place, you sat where the waiter put you, and the food was very limited.

There was one financial puzzle that I could never work out. A notice outside the dining room stated that the cost of a meal was 2,000 escudos, however, if you decided not to eat in the dining room and opted for a meal in the grill bar, the hotel would give you 500 escudos towards your meal in the grill bar, which would cost considerably more than 2,000. I had the feeling that they were gaining on me somewhere.

On asking our courier about the food she said that all these things were cut down to such fine profit margins that their tour company wasn't even going to send tourists to this particular hotel that winter, which was a terrible shame. It was superbly equipped, the Portuguese were their usual charming selves, but of course they had to make a profit.

But the setting, a beautiful ascending staircase as you came in the main gateway, lovely pillared landings, great deep armchairs in scattered lounges, pleasant bars — really first-class food was meant to go with these surroundings.

We did eat out a couple of times, which proved inexpensive and certainly better than the hotel fare. However, the food in the grill bar was superb.

There was a regular bus service to a beach ten minutes away where there were miles and miles of sand and for a very small sum you could hire a sun shade. The hotel also had its own swimming pool and restaurant there.

What amazed us was that the beach was empty, at most there were half a dozen people sitting on it, so it worked out to about two miles each. The water was warm, the swimming was good, but when you went past the wooden palings to get into the enclosure where the swimming pool and restaurant were, perhaps because it was Portugal, the people there looked as if they were in a sardine tin. There were probably a couple of hundred oiled bodies lying side by side, taking up every inch of space around the pool, and a dozen people actually in the pool itself. There was a very good restaurant at the side where inexpensively you could buy anything from a sandwich to a five-course meal, with wine, beers, the lot. It really was lovely.

I tried to reason out why everyone stuck round the pool and didn't go into the sea. I thought: well, I was young once, and I wanted to be where the crumpet was; but when I looked at the pool, quite a number of the people there were rather large ladies of the older age group wearing bikinis that were gestures rather than pieces of wearing apparel — not a pretty sight.

Lagos was a lovely little town. With its monument of Henry the Navigator on the sea front it was one of the places where it was thought he might have had his school of navigation, certainly the

Governor's Palace was his headquarters.

It was a nice place to wander around. We went to the small unmarked arcade, a white two-storeyed building, where the first slave auctions used to be held. There is the delightful St Anthony's Chapel with its carvings, beautiful altar, and on the floor, the tomb of an Irishman, Hugh Beatty, who was something to do with the Portuguese army in the eighteenth century. We visited the museum, the brewery, but enjoyed more strolling around the streets and shops which were often cool, shaded by tall buildings either side, with restaurants setting tables all the way down the middle of the street.

As far as I could see, the whole of the population of Lagos lived on a diet of grilled sardines. There were plenty of good bistros and bars to eat and drink in. It was not as big a town or quite as interesting a town as Faro, but a pleasant town and there's something about towns that makes them so much nicer than resorts. You felt that you were in Portugal and there were local people earning a living all around you; you weren't as yet in a faceless, concrete jungle as so many places in the sun are becoming.

Happily, the Portuguese, unlike the Spanish, are determined not to be taken over by the British and are now pulling down all English signs offering fish and chips, cream teas, etc., and replacing them with Portuguese equivalents.

We went for a coach trip into the mountains to see a most spectacular view, staying for a time and going round the old city of Silves. When the Moors occupied the Algarve in the eighth century, Silves was the capital, and their headquarters. Over the years the rivers leading to the sea have become silted up, but in those days Silves was a very important port and an almost impregnable castle was built on top of a hill. It wasn't until the middle of the thirteenth century that the Portuguese actually captured and threw out the Moors for good, and later transferred the capital of the Algarve from there to Faro, where it remains today.

There is an extremely well preserved castle and lovely cathedral adjoining it in the midst of this beautiful countryside.

Our day trip to the mountains was marred by the fact that we were two hours picking people up from other hotels on the way up and two hours dropping them off on the way back and, of course, we had several obligatory stops at various gift shops.

In spite of all that, we had a lovely day. The view for miles from the top of the mountains and certainly Silves were well worth a visit — you can't have everything.

This applied to our hotel and its food. The hotel was superb, the food was moderate with a very limited selection. You queued and were shown to a different place each evening which you shared with another couple.

We were lucky that all the people we met were nice; a few were quite fascinating.

The first couple were the Maguires. He was a salesman for an electronics company and she a nurse at a private nursing home. We saw quite a lot of Pat and Joy whilst we were there, going to the beach with them several times. They had some great stories to tell.

Pat was an Irish Roman Catholic from Belfast and obviously had been a bit of a wild lad in his younger days, and Joy was English and Protestant. The couple had met in England and had been going out together for some time when, though almost penniless, they decided to get engaged. They felt that Pat's parents in Ireland should be informed and that Pat should go home and tell them personally.

They clubbed together all the money they had, which would just pay the fare to Belfast, and Joy was set to have a few days on her own.

On the first day she bumped into her father, a poet who wandered in and out of their lives. On finding that Pat had gone to Ireland on his own because they hadn't enough money for them both to go, he produced money for an air ticket for Joy. She would be able to catch up with Pat and meet his thirteen brothers and sisters and his parents when he broke the news to them about his engagement to an English Protestant.

She had her hair done in a beehive, put her best silver fox fur round her neck (she'd bought it at an Oxfam shop), and set off for Belfast, tracking down Pat's address, eventually finding the right street and at last the right house.

She knocked on the door. A dark-haired young girl answered.

'I'm Pat's girlfriend,' said Joy.

'Which one?' said the girl.

This put Joy back a bit. 'Well,' she said, 'could I come in and see him?'

'I'm afraid you can't,' said the girl. 'He's in England.'

Pat had never made it to Ireland. With the money for his air fare in his pocket he'd bumped into somebody with whom he'd done his national service. They'd gone off to have one drink and by the time they'd finished reminiscing, he had no money left for his fare. He daren't go and face Joy.

Joy was eventually invited in and had to inform the family that she was Pat's fiancée. Eventually it all got sorted and they later got married and had children: but Pat's mother, Joy said, always used to say, 'You've never looked as smart as that day you first arrived with your beehive hair-do and your fox fur round your neck, on a warm summer's day.'

The other couple with whom we became friendly were an older couple from Canada, Ken and Louise Edmondson, who were wandering around Europe. He was a strapping great man in his late sixties; a hunting, shooting, fishing man who had a farm out in the wilds in Canada somewhere. I could sit and listen to him for hours.

The stories I liked best were his Alaskan ones. He used to be taken fishing and shooting in deepest Alaska by Jack, a Canadian with the strangest accent, who was married to an Eskimo woman. Ken would tell tales of catching salmon and shooting caribou, but his stories of Jack and his Eskimo wife were the most interesting of all.

Jack used to say that his Eskimo wife literally kept him alive.

They needed to shoot twelve caribou to see them through the winter, and they'd go off to hunt them on their snow scooter. Sometimes a white-out (blizzard) would spring up and they would have to take shelter, or die. They would put the snow scooter on its side, the Eskimo wife would lay several caribou skins fur upwards on the snow by the scooter, then she and Jack would lie under another pile of caribou skins with the fur facing down. The snow would cover them and when it stopped snowing they would dig themselves out and in this way she kept them both alive.

Whilst Ken and his friends were out fishing with Jack, ever resourceful she would be busily bottling the fish they caught to store away for the winter.

Another of Ken's tales about Jack, this great brawny man of the wild, went thus.

One summer Jack had been fooling around with one or two other women in the encampment that they came to in the summer. They had a house built there, properly equipped with windows, doors, plumbing and other conveniences. This took a great deal of capital outlay as everything had to be brought from so far away.

One day after Jack had been at his shenanigans, his wife said, 'When the pilot comes from Winnipeg, will you ask him to bring me a bottle of gin?'

After the next trip to Winnipeg, the pilot duly delivered a bottle of gin.

Up to this stage Jack's wife had not mentioned anything about his extra-marital activities. She took the bottle of gin in her hand, sat down in the room with him, took a few slurps from the bottle and for the first time tackled the subject. 'I'm displeased with you,' she said, and took a few more slurps from her bottle. She added, 'In fact, I'm very displeased with you. You've been fooling around with women. You've disgraced our family name. You've made me look foolish. I'm very, very displeased with you.' She took two more slurps of gin then picked up a chair and systematically went round the house smashing every single window, knowing that the glass replacements would have to come 1,800 miles from Winnipeg. Mission accomplished she sat down, had one more gin and that was the end of the matter.

Whether he ever misbehaved again, Ken said he never knew, but they remained together. He said, 'But I did ask him about his accent. There was something odd about it; it wasn't true Canadian.' It's always difficult asking people about their accents, so Ken put it as tactfully as he could. 'Where do you hail from originally, Jack?' he said to this big Canadian trapper.

'Wolverhampton,' said Jack, and proffered no further information.

I wondered by what routes he had travelled from Wolverhampton to an isolated Eskimo settlement in north Alaska.

Another couple we sat next to one night had a daughter that once nearly became engaged to Ron Dickinson, our junior partner in Tadchester, and one night (I knew it as soon as we sat down) the couple sharing our table were a doctor and his wife from Bristol and, of course, we knew people who knew people who knew people.

All in all it was a very good holiday. The Portuguese are lovely, Portugal is lovely, there's sunshine, golden beaches and I think they're already taking steps to see it's not going to be spoilt. I expect it's because I'm getting old that I like towns rather than resorts. If I was twenty or twenty-one I expect all I would want would be sea, sun, girls and drinks. Historic places and views could always be saved for later years.

But the turmoil at the airport and an unpleasant train ride very late at night, rather put us off package holidays. The train was certainly the dirtiest, shabbiest train I've ever been on.

I noticed in each compartment an arrow indicating the way to the luggage compartment for air travellers. Each arrow ended up at a toilet. I could see some very confused foreigners getting on this train.

It was so bad I wrote to British Rail about it, who apologised and said it was a train they were hoping to replace in the future.

Although we had had a good holiday in a very pleasant place, we thought afterwards how much easier it is to pop all your things in the back of the car and nip across the Channel to explore France which, along with outings on the Thames, was one of our great loves. And there was more of France left for me to explore than I could cover in a lifetime.

6

Lucky For Some

I FIRST met Robin Treaton on a disastrous Moroccan holiday when about fifty of us had a fortnight's tour through Morocco in a coach, staying in some frightful places, everybody being ill and nearly being lynched by the locals.

Friends you meet on holiday always swear to keep in touch, and it seldom happens. Robin Treaton was an exception. He has remained a friend ever since, and it must be at least ten years since we set out on this ill-fated expedition.

We became buddies during this trip, standing out from the rest — we were different from them. Not that we had any special talents but when we met the other members of the expedition we found, and this wasn't clear in the brochure, that this was a holiday for the under thirty-fives, and at the time Robin was forty-seven and I was fifty-three. We were practically geriatric compared with the rest, but we certainly held our own with the other males in the party, and even excelled ourselves on occasions such as when the eccentric Robin suddenly decided at 3 a.m. that the offensive toilet at this particular camp site at which we were staying needed cleaning out, and armed with palm branches he dragged me down to unblock these holes in the ground. That, plus a few buckets of water, made morning ablutions less offensive to the rest of the party.

I can quite believe Robin's story of when he was in Bangkok. Being at a loose end one evening he hired a rickshaw, and decided, under the direction of the rickshaw puller, to undertake a tour of the town's drinking establishments. Although drinking was not one of Robin's main interests, certainly not the main one, when he did sit down to drink he was one of these hollow-legged people who could drink vast quantities of alcohol without it having any great effect on him.

On this occasion they visited about ten establishments, and, defying local custom, Robin insisted that the rickshaw puller join him glass for glass on this glorified pub crawl. After twelve stops Robin was just getting into his stride, but the rickshaw puller, who probably hadn't had a square meal for a month, and was watching just about a year's wages going on drink, was out for the count. There was nothing for it other than for Robin to bodily carry his driver, dump him in his own rickshaw, get between the pulling shafts himself, and tow the chap back as far as his hotel. They had travelled further than Robin had estimated. It took him a good two hours to pull the chap along, by which time Robin was just about physically out on his feet, and the rickshaw puller sufficiently recovered to demand a fee from Robin for the evening's work.

A typical card arrived one day from Robin, who was in Turkey, to say, 'A little boy asked me if I would like a virgin. I asked him if it was his sister. "No," he said, "it's my mother."'

Robin was no Errol Flynn but was not far behind him in his success with the opposite sex. He wasn't the dashing swash-buckling type — in fact, he was almost a deadringer for Eddie 'the Eagle' Edwards of Olympic ski-jumping fame.

He resembled him facially, and seemed to have many of his mannerisms, and, as with Eddie the Eagle, they endeared him to everyone.

For many years Robin was unmarried though he always talked about his ex, which was a prolonged unmarried time with one particular lady who in the end married someone else. Although, even so he spent a lot of time with her and her new mate.

He was not really the marrying sort.

He was an engineer in a large aeronautical works in Birmingham. Part of his work necessitated travelling down to the west of England and often he would call in and stay with us.

He came on several boating trips, usually the short ones, and was very handy if the propeller got stuck. I remember our first trip with him: half the time he was diving under the boat unwinding something that had got stuck round the propeller shaft.

He drove a long green sporty-looking car of indeterminate age; it was always immaculate. He always meant to change it but could never afford to, mainly because all his money went on travel.

Robin went everywhere, South America, North America, India, Thailand, Nepal, Australia, and whereas most people who came back from these exotic places had stories of magnificent temples or ancient ruins, Robin would talk about the various conquests he'd made on each trip, and I would listen in envy and half belief.

He led a fairly hairy sort of life and many of the ladies he conquered on holiday had big hairy boyfriends at home, one or two of whom rang up and threatened him. Some of the ladies who went on these trips forgot to put on their wedding rings and when he came back he sometimes found there were unexpected husbands in the background who weren't always too pleased to see him.

Whatever he did he was always successful. There was something very appealing about him, just in the way you see Eddie Edwards stuffing newspaper into boots three sizes too big for him, competing against East Germans who'd been picked out as children and trained in army camps 24 hours a day to compete against the true amateurs of the world. Robin gave you this same warmhearted amateur, British feeling. But Robin, unlike Eddie the Eagle, rarely came last.

He came back disconsolate from a trip up the Nile. For once he'd been unsuccessful and for once he'd really liked somebody very much. He'd fallen for an American girl who, at the end of the trip, went back to her homeland, and America is much more difficult to commute to from Birmingham than is, say, Solihull or even London, so he had to pursue her from a distance.

Robin called this his 'lucky' year.

It began when somebody crashed into his car in a car park and went off without leaving a name and address, resulting in several hundred pounds' worth of repairs.

The next 'lucky' event happened when Robin was driving along the motorway one day. Suddenly he noticed a bouncing metal ingot coming over the barrier. By ducking just in time and pulling towards the hard shoulder the ingot smashed into the windscreen cutting into his right hand rather than his head. He could very easily have been killed.

A following motorist summoned an ambulance and all the emergency services; Robin was able to climb out of his car but he'd badly damaged his hand and, in fact, it never ever got completely better. What annoyed him most were the comments he received from everyone who attended him: 'My God, you were lucky.'

In a way he was; the ingot could have killed him but he felt that he was rather unlucky that it was *his* car that an unidentified object had collided with.

When he arrived at the hospital, they stitched him up, heard his story, and again they said how lucky he was.

Where he was definitely unlucky was that the police could not trace the owner of the ingot, so he got no compensation or insurance for the damage done to his car or the injury done to his person.

Robin did wonder from time to time what you had to do to be unlucky.

Eventually his luck did seem to change. He had continued to correspond with the American lady he'd failed to conquer and she, perhaps through some dull American winter, decided Robin wasn't so bad after all and agreed to come to Europe and go on a holiday with him to Portugal.

These were definite signs of surrender. She had left all the bookings to him. He hired a car for a week and rented a villa.

The American lady arrived. They had a couple of free days before they went to their villa.

They picked up the car from the airport and set off to a beautiful luxurious hotel that Robin had picked out in the hills above Lisbon.

This was the night they were at last going to consummate their friendship, and they were going to do it in style.

The hotel was absolutely magnificent and surprisingly, not very expensive. The room had a huge four-poster bed, from which he could hardly keep his eyes. It had an en-suite lounge, a splendid bathroom with a toilet like a throne and a great high-walled bath, which was difficult to step out of. It all looked too good to be true. They were both tired and hot, sweaty and dirty after their travelling, so the first call was for a long, cool drink. Champagne was duly brought to the room. A plunge in the glorious bath was the next order of the day.

The American girl went first. He could hear her splashing around and singing, which was a good prelude as she knew a fate worse than death awaited her.

Eventually she came out in a tartan dressing gown and said, 'Well, I'll get into something comfortable whilst you go and have your bath.'

Robin, who had been busy exploring the room, had already uncovered a black negligée — this was going to be the night of nights. It was already early evening, but food and drink could wait till later.

He filled the bath and then wallowed in it with scented oils, in no hurry — everything was going to be just perfect. He stood up in the bath, half dried himself and took a step over the high bath wall. He put his foot straight down on a piece of soap, slipped, and skidded across the bathroom floor. There was a searing pain in the area of his nether regions and blood started to pour all over the floor. He shouted with pain as he slid, tearing something, he wasn't quite sure what. Hearing the shouts his girlfriend, now in a black, see-through neligée, came in to find the man of the moment lying naked on the floor in a pool of blood. She screamed.

A jagged tile edge had caused a seven-inch cut in his scrotum. It was bleeding profusely. They rang the desk for help; the assistant manager came up. In this particular Portuguese hotel nobody understood very much English, particularly the word for scrotum, but by various hand sign language the assistant manager suggested he went to the hospital, which fortunately was only about three hundred yards away.

To stop the bleeding Robin and his girlfriend put a couple of towels on him like nappies and managed to pull his trousers over the top. Dressed thus he waddled off to the hospital where, thank goodness, the doctor spoke good English.

He looked down at Robin's injury. 'My God, you've been lucky,' he said. He didn't realise how near he'd come to Robin inflicting him with some grievous bodily harm.

He was stitched up under local anaesthetic, had various plasters and things stuck on the wound and was advised to go to a clinic near the villa they'd booked, to have his stitches out in about seven days' time. Once more as they were leaving the hospital the doctor patted him on the shoulder. 'You're a lucky man,' he said. 'It could have been much worse.'

The injury prevented any consummation of friendship but the pair made the best of their holiday, and had a smashing time in good weather, touring round northern Portugal, reporting to the clinic to have his stitches out. Very often a blow to the area where Robin had received his injury causes bleeding and swelling of the scrotum. Many men who have had vasectomies have staggered into the surgery with dangling lumps the size and shape of footballs.

Robin was fortunate that this hadn't occurred to him.

This fact was also observed by the clinic doctors, who were Swedish, for some reason doing a spell in Portugal. Their first comments were, 'You've been very lucky', little realising that they were putting their lives in peril.

This chaste holiday seemed to have done Robin and his American friend, Pearl, good. In his mid-fifties, for the first time Robin had been conquered. Pam and I went up to Birmingham six months later to a registry office wedding and Robin, the oldest swinger in town, had eventually met his match.

They had a flat for a short time and acquired a dog, and then bought half a house in the country that dated back to the time of William and Conqueror, the other half being occupied by a delightful couple with two small children.

There was a communal garden and was one slight problem: the children had a rabbit and Robin and Pearl had a dog. If they were careful and the children let them know when the rabbit was going to have a run (and anyway the dog didn't seem particularly interested in rabbits), they shouldn't have any problems.

Months went by and, even though they were in two separate halves of the same house, they saw very little of their neighbours.

To their horror, one dark night, in

came the dog dragging a very dead rabbit.

They didn't know what to do. The rabbit looked a bit wet but didn't seem to have been too mangled. They got out the hair dryer, washed it, dried it and once all its fur was fluffy and clean there was no obvious injury.

Robin and Pearl were in a quandary.

'I know,' said Robin. 'Let's put it back in the hutch.'

They crept out quietly in the dark and from behind bushes, opened the hutch, which to their surprise was shut, and popped in the rabbit.

All was well until the next morning when they heard a sudden hysterical screaming and a knocking from the lady next door.

'The rabbit's back in his hutch,' screamed the neighbour.

'Well, shouldn't it be in its hutch?' asked Robin.

'No,' said the near-frantic woman. 'The rabbit died two weeks ago. We buried it.'

They calmed her down, pleading ignorance of the whole event, and agreeing with their neighbour that some supernatural force had been at work. Then they helped re-bury the rabbit.

Alone at last Robin turned to Pearl and said, 'I guess this is just the beginning of another lucky day for me.'

7

Neither a Lender nor a Borrower Be

PART of the fun of having a boat was lending it to family and friends who were either having a holiday for the first time, or who were so broke they couldn't afford to go anywhere else.

I knew when I lent it to Jonathan next door that it would be in good hands. Jonathan, his father and brother are engineer mechanics of the highest order, and if I glanced from my balcony to the drive next door any weekend, I could almost guarantee that if Jonathan wasn't taking the engine out of his car, he was at least putting it back.

After a week on the boat with friends, Jonathan returned it, gleaming clean as it had never been before, with the engine purring like a kitten.

I do not have the same confidence in my own family: none of us know one end of a spanner from another.

It was with some trepidation that I saw Trevor, Jane and two friends, Fred and another Jane, sailing off into the gloaming. Before they set off I had pinned a set of instructions to the back of the cabin door, and put a lock and chain in Trevor's hand saying, 'If you moor in Oxford or Henley for the night, chain the boat to one of the fixed rings on the towpath.' Unfortunately vandalism has reached our river banks, and some yobbos delight in cutting the moorings of boats at night and pushing the craft out into the stream. There is no doubt that if they haven't already done so, one day they would kill someone. I would rank the cutting of moorings of occupied boats as attempted manslaughter, and would impose the requisite penalty.

Trevor reached Oxford safely but rang from there to say the battery was flat and they couldn't start the engine. This surprised me: you have to use an awful lot of juice to flatten one of those batteries. They had also had an adventure. They had been playing cards when they heard a knocking on the side of the boat. They lifted the cabin flap to find a man in a punt asking them politely if they realised they were drifting downstream. Someone had cut their moorings.

The punt man kindly manoeuvred them back to their mooring, and Trevor belatedly chained the boat to the bank. Without the kindly intervention of the man in the punt, they could have had a tragic end to their holiday.

'What time was this?' I enquired.

'About 2 a.m.,' said Trevor.

I then realised that if they had had electricity burning till 2 a.m., there was every reason to have a flat battery.

Trevor went to the nearest garage and bought a new car battery. This was enough to get them going, but I doubted if it would be man enough for all the electrical equipment on the boat, so I decided to intercept them at the Rose Revived at Newbridge, and take off the main boat battery and bring it home to be charged.

As I thought, there was a call from the Rose Revived the next morning. Flat battery again. I took out the newly charged main battery and saw them get started up. Thankfully I also saw the sun come out; it had rained steadily for the whole of the holiday up to now, and the morale of the crew was low.

This was the turning point, from then on they had a splendid time — the sun blazed down, no more mechanical or battery troubles, and they chained themselves to quays both in Oxford and Henley. Paul, Gill and Daisy May came over on their last day. We had a rough idea where they would be, so met up with them below Goring Lock.

Paul, Gill and Daisy May joined them for the last few miles, whilst Pam and I went back to prepare hot baths and arrange a barbecue in the garden.

They brought a spotless boat into our mooring like seasoned sailors. Who knows, given time we might all become mechanics.

The next borrowing was by my godson, Tim, who was taking a mixed crew of old school friends. Their start was delayed by one lady crew member, who, when she arrived, looked as if she would be more at home at Ascot rather than on a river boat, and had caught a train to Wallington only to discover she couldn't find a river there and thought she should try Wallingford.

The main disaster on their holiday was to get a mooring rope entangled around the propeller shaft. It took three boys a whole afternoon's diving to clear it, but that's messing about in boats for you.

Tim is a delightful young man, he stayed the night with us after his week, and I had to listen patiently to him regarding all his affairs of the heart. He was in desperate need of advice. I gave him the following article which I had written many years ago as a medical student.

How to Choose Your Mate
Anatomically the best wives are stocky, wide hipped, thick waisted, full chested members of the female sex, with short strong fingers, powerful backs, tremendous stamina and of the intellect that wouldn't waste £1 on the housekeeping that could just as easily be spent on beer and fags. With this in mind the average male will look for the slimmest,

fragile, most expensive looking bird he can find. The main factors influencing his decision being the size, mobility and shape of the soft tissue swellings on the front of the female thorax (chest), and the length, curvature, muscle balance of the trunk body supports (the legs). The main vote going in a ratio of three to two to the legs, or under-carriage.

From then on the rules are simple:

Pursue the bird object of your desire for forty-eight hours. Then stop. If you go beyond this time period she will lose all interest as she will think she has got you. She'll put it down in her book as another conquest and then devote her time to trying to pick up her best friend's boy who is an inch shorter than her but has never looked at her.

After the initial forty-eight hours you start paying attention to the object bird's best friend, who has a pleasant face but whose under-carriage doesn't fill your desired specification.

This changes your bird from being on the point of giving you up to deciding that you are all she ever wanted and she will fling herself at your feet;

thus changing her from the austere, wonderful, unapproachable beauty that you were first attracted to, to something available and humiliatingly easy that you immediately lose interest in.

As her friend, who you have been chatting up (in spite of her bad legs), shows no reciprocal interest, as she has just become engaged, you find her the most irresistible female you have ever seen, and if she marries this chap who has swinishly tricked her into wearing his ring, life will hold nothing for you and you will apply for a job as a porter in Albert Schweitzer's leper colony.

If she is fool enough to break off her engagement for you, forty-eight hours after the initial victory, she will fall into the same category as the first bird and you will realise how mad you were to have considered having anything to do with a bird with legs like hers.

Your first bird will then have got over her disappointment with you and have paired off with some other swine, and immediately will recapture all her old allure.

You will then fling yourself at her,

but you being now so available, become less attractive, as well as her remembering the last time. She won't have anything to do with you, unless of course you start chatting up her second best friend, then the whole cycle will repeat itself.

These permutations are great fun for a few years, but if by the age of seventy-five you have not broken the cycle, even though the citations of individual cases will prove me wrong, it is unlikely that this article will be of much use to you.

If you were able to remember back to the alluring stage, when a bird is humiliating herself at your feet, then it would be possible to actually pick for your own which ever bird you really wanted, but of course it never works out like this.

The best thing is to marry the girl next door if she will have you, as there is no doubt it's the birds who decide on who is going to be their mate; the average man has no say in the matter at all.

Tim read the article, then looked up thoughtfully.

'But, Uncle Bob,' he said, 'there aren't any girls next door.'

'Well, Tim,' I said, 'it will have to be girl next-door-but-one.'

8

An Act of Doc

I HAD spent most of my working life in Tadchester.

Tadchester is a market town with a rising population of about 8,000. It stands on the estuary of the River Tad in one of the most beautiful parts of the Somerset coast, with the resorts of Sandford-on-Sea and Stowin nearby. Although primarily a market town, it still has some fishing, an increasing amount of light industry and a small mine that produces pigments, a residue from the time when the main industry in the town was coal-mining.

We were the only general practice in the town, and when I first arrived, the senior partner was the beloved Steve Maxwell, who had a special interest in medicine, the bluff Henry Johnson, the surgeon of the practice, was the second partner, and Jack Hart, who gave most of the anaesthetics, batted at number three.

I joined as number four, and most of the midwifery came my way. In later years we engaged a fifth partner, Ron Dickinson, who took a keen interest in E.N.T.s and an even greater interest in running, jumping, squash, sailing and water-skiing. He was always bouncing about doing something physical, a sort of cross between Peter Pan and Tigger from *Winnie The Pooh*.

Later on, when I was off work for some months, we had a locum, Catherine Carlton, a dentist's wife. When I returned to work, we kept her on as a half-time partner.

How quickly the years pass by. I remember when I went to be interviewed for the practice vacancy in 1955. I thought then that Steve Maxwell and Henry Johnson were old men, and that Jack Hart was late middle-aged. In fact, Steve and Henry must have been in their mid-forties and Jack Hart about thirty-five. Now, sadly, Steve Maxwell and Henry Johnson are dead, Jack Hart has retired and I have retired to Wallingford. It is unbelievable to think that Ron Dickinson, now the senior partner, is fast approaching retirement age himself.

Since we've moved to Wallingford we've seen a lot of Ron and his wife Annette. They frequently come to stay and Ron hasn't changed or aged a bit. As soon as they arrive Ron changes into a pink tracksuit and goes bouncing off down the towpath for a couple of miles, then runs back, has a quick hot bath and dashes off to the nearest pub. After downing a couple of pints of draught bitter he is at last fit to face us and the evening. By the time we approach the small hours, he has usually divested himself of most of his clothes and sits grinning like a pixie in his underpants with a large glass of port in his hand. There is certainly never a dull moment when Ron is around.

We have become a popular stopping-off place for all and sundry coming up from the West Country, being near to both London and Heathrow; often friends leave their cars with us while they visit the big city or fly abroad.

Several have come on the boat with us — Pam and Bill Law, Eric, Zara and Nicholas — but, one trip I was really looking forward to was with my old friend Chris Parfitt (C.P.), the editor of the *Tadchester Gazette*. It was to be a combined fishing-cum-boating holiday with C.P. as crew and me as captain and chief cook.

We had had an unforgettable holiday together before, *en famille*, eight of us in France and I hoped this boat trip would be as successful.

Sadly, although it wasn't a bad holiday, it wasn't as good as I had hoped. C.P. was not as river-wise as I had expected — he wasn't desperately good in locks, or at jumping out to moor the boat — and in the end C.P. developed some mysterious stomach upset and we had to return to base early. I had quite forgotten that most of C.P.'s river experience was derived from sitting on the bank, under a green umbrella, pipe clenched firmly in his mouth, dreaming of the pint of beer he was going to drink at the end of the day's activities.

It was lovely seeing him, even for a short time, and happily he perked up when we got home and Pam took over the catering.

I used to take the fishing magazine in which C.P. wrote a weekly humorous philosophical column, supposedly on fishing. In fact it could be on anything from the Pope to tiddlywinks. I thought he was the wittiest writer in print.

On reading his column some months after our holiday, I realised its contents were C.P.'s side of our trip together. The article went as follows.

An Act of Doc

'There's an insurance man in the paper,' I said to Dearly Beloved across the breakfast table, 'who reckons that the average husband is worth £500,000.'

'Really?' she said, looking at me in my morning glory. 'I'll take 50p for cash.'

Some people . . .

On the way to work, I read of a fifteen-year-old Italian lad, the world champion table-soccer player, whose right index finger — the one he flicks with — is insured for £25,000.

Gad, I thought. If a little lad's index finger is worth that much just for flicking some plastic footballers about, what must mine be worth? Where would I be without its aid on the bank for such essential operations as taking the ring off a can, guiding the hook into a pinkie and out of a perchie?

Shock horror at the office. Phone call from Dave Bogart, the hunky American person and former demon angler of Upper Black Eddy on the Delaware. Dave couldn't come to work on account of he was on his way home the night before and he fell over a bloke who was cleaning his car in the dark. Broke both arms.

With both arms in plaster Dave would be in no condition for several weeks even to bait up, let alone cast out.

I'd better get myself insured, I thought, before something terrible happens. No use any longer relying on my lucky socks, rabbit's foot or Fozzie Bear mascot to keep me out of the old emergency ward.

The trouble with angling, though, is that accidents are seldom straight-forward. And it's rarely the likely one which gets you. Take my last trip out with Doc Thumper [my pen name], physician extraordinary and skipper of the luxury 27 foot *Sea Grey*.

Up the Thames we went, along the narrower upper reaches, as is our wont. We came to a lock, the keeper of which was away for din-dins.

'I'll operate the gates,' said Doc. 'And you can stay in charge of the boat.'

'Aye aye, Cap'n,' I said. 'Have no fear. Old Longjohn Parfitt'll see ee roight. Oh arr . . . '

'On second thoughts,' said Doc, 'I'll stay on board the boat. You work the gates. Sure you know how to do it?'

'Easy peasy Cap'n,' said I. I leapt on the towpath, tied a rope around one of those bollard things and opened the first gate.

Fired with enthusiasm, I ran up to the next set of gates and started winching away.

'Help!' cried Doc, as about twenty miles of Thames water started moving down towards him. 'You're supposed to close the other one first! And I'm supposed to be inside the lock!'

'What's keeping you?' I hollered, winching madly in reverse.

'Those twelve granny knots you tied around the bollard. Are you sure you've done this before?'

A bit further upstream it was Doc's turn to make a boo-boo. We passed an island in midstream. On the other side of the island, and running to the far bank, was a weir.

Once past the island, Doc said, 'There's a lovely little creek behind the weir, and I know an old lady who lives along there. She'll let us fish from the bottom of her garden.'

So saying, he swung the boat hard-a-starboard (who says I know nowt about it?) round the back of the island, and headed for the creek. The current was flowing strongly and we found ourselves moving swiftly towards the weir.

'Soon be there,' said Doc.

'Oh, what's it say on that board sticking out of the water?' he said.

'D-A-N-G-E-R . . . danger,' I said

(as in 'banger'). My mind must have been on something else. 'No! Oh-my-gawd! It's DANGER! As in 'ranger'!'

'As in what?' shouted Doc over the noise of the engine.

'Ranger! As in Lone Ranger! Tonto! Hi-yo Silver . . . away!'

'This is no time to be playing cowboys,' shouted Doc. 'I think we might be in some small difficulty here . . .'

By a combination of skilful seamanship and pure fluke, Doc turned the boat around then guided it painfully upstream out of the fast water. The old lady up the creek could wait for another day.

Some time later we approached a couple of small bays on the left bank.

'This looks fine,' said Doc. 'We'll moor here.'

I crouched on the bows like a tar to the manner born, mooring rope in hand, and leapt on to the bank as we entered the first bay. The boat kept on going and dragged me halfway down the bank before I could let go and cling on to a handy tree.

'Why the hell didn't you stop?' I shouted.

'I meant the second bay,' said Doc. 'Now stop messing about in that tree and make yourself useful.'

The useful bit was to moor the boat. Doc threw up a couple of iron spikes which just missed my vitals, and a two-pound hammer which landed neatly on my foot.

'I'm getting a bit fed up with this,' I said.

'Not to worry,' said Doc. 'We're here now. Tell you what, while you're tacking up I'll cook us a lovely mixed grill on the stove.'

Now do you see all the possibilities for accident on that one innocent trip out? The boat could have been turned over or washed away by the rush of lock water; it could have been swept over the weir; I would have had a ducking if it had not been for the handy tree; I just missed being speared by the mooring spikes and was actually struck a deadly blow on the big toe by the two-pound hammer. Bang would have gone the no-claims bonus. But it wasn't any of those that did the damage.

That night, both Doc and I were assailed by fearsome indigestion and drove each other potty by groaning until the small hours. Now that was the real hazard of the trip yet it probably wouldn't have been covered by insurance. It wasn't so much an act of God as an act of Doc.

Have you ever tried his cooking?

I rang C.P. after I had read it, swearing that I would never cook for him again.

'Put that in writing,' said C.P., 'and we are friends for life.'

C.P. was a true fisherman, and on the river it was always a bit fisherman versus boats, and crewing on a boat rather divided his loyalties.

Though C.P. and his wife often came to stay and C.P. was quite happy to fish from the end of the garden, I could never entice him back on board again, even though I promised not to cook.

9

On the Air

IN 1961 I sent my first unsolicited script off to the Talks Department of the BBC. My story was about two old ladies, one of whom had been bedridden for forty-seven years and how this lady had made a great success of her life, confined as she was.

My script was accepted and I went to Exeter and recorded it. Not only was it broadcast on *Woman's Hour*, but it was repeated. For this to happen in Tadchester was fame indeed and I grew at least six inches in stature overnight.

One mistake I made in my broadcast was to disguise the identities of the two ladies. I called them Miss Gill and Miss Booth, whereas their names were Miss Oake and Miss Lord, and many of their friends throughout England (and they had a wide number of people with whom they corresponded), recognised them. What I hadn't realised was that my broadcast would open up their world as it did. They became overnight celebrities and if I'd called them by their proper names, they would have been more famous still.

In the story the bedridden lady said, 'People come to me because I have time to listen.' And it became a catch phrase that people remembered.

Heady with success I sent my second script off to the BBC. This was about a man who knew he was going to die and who died on the exact day he was told he was going to, and it made quite a moving story.

Again the BBC accepted it and this time I went to Plymouth to record it. I wasn't very good at reading from scripts and it took two hours to record. I could talk well but I couldn't read scripts — you need to be an actor. It was interesting that the producer of this particular talk went down with stomach ulcers a couple of weeks after having to cope with me!

But again, like the first story, the BBC not only broadcast it once, but repeated it.

In Tadchester I was absolutely famous. People nodded to me in the street, happy to know me; even my partners looked at me with a sort of new-found respect.

Back in 1961 radio was very important. People listened to it just as much as they watched television.

After these successes I realised that anything I sent to the BBC would automatically be taken and broadcast — I was a natural. Unfortunately the next twenty-seven scripts I sent in were rejected.

In between the time of my second successful broadcast and before my rejections started to arrive, somebody from Tadchester told me that a friend of theirs was about to give a broadcast on Radio Bristol. Would I, with all my experience, i.e. six minutes on *Woman's Hour*, help?

I was, of course, very happy to help any struggling star who hadn't made it to the top as I had, and my friend Eric from the Tadchester Radio Services lent me a tape-recorder — even tape-recorders were rare in those days — and I suggested that this potential lady broadcaster should record her broadcast and listen to herself. I also volunteered to listen to the tape and said I would be happy to give an opinion.

I listened to it and thought it was terrible.

The lady had a broad Devon accent and her talk concerned her husband, the lodgers they had at their guesthouse and the pigs on their farm.

Obviously not in my league.

I kept my thoughts to myself, told her it was very good and wished her luck, thinking it a pity she hadn't a golden voice like mine — poor lass. I knew she would never broadcast again.

This broadcast was the first of many hundreds she made for *Woman's Hour* at the BBC. She became a household name and the BBC made several records of her collective broadcasts for general release.

She was about five hundred times more successful than I was!

I soldiered on, sending out broadcasting scripts and having one or two more accepted. Then, because I was a doctor, I drifted into giving medical broadcasts, mainly involving the answering of medical questions.

It was very convenient. If I was going up to London for any reason, I would ring up *Woman's Hour* and ask whether there were any medical questions that needed answering, and very often they would fit me in for a recording, which paid my fare.

I also continued to have some success with submitted scripts.

One, which I felt was better than most, was quite a moving story of a man who had spent ten years of his life trying to get a play put on in the West End. He was actually our landlord when we'd lived in a flat in a big house; he'd lived in a room upstairs.

I sent it to the people at the BBC I'd been working with, and they sent it back, not with a normal letter but with a rejection slip. So I sent it to Radio Bristol, who accepted it, and it was put on the Rolfe Whiteman show.

What I didn't know was that the Rolfe Whiteman show that afternoon was going to be part of *Woman's Hour*, so it got on *Woman's Hour* after all.

Rolfe Whiteman was a very famous broadcaster. I once said on a radio programme that he had a voice that sounded as if he'd been gargling with Devon cream. This gave rise to a lot of angry letters and 'phone calls saying that he was a Wiltshire man and I'd inferred he'd come from Devon. I don't know whether they make cream in Wiltshire.

My broadcast about the man upstairs, which I had to read from a script, was made from the Bristol studios.

It was very poignant. This delightful man whom we knew well, had isolated himself for ten years, writing away at his plays and also keeping himself available so that if a film or theatre company needed him he could be off, literally within 24 hours' notice, anywhere in the world.

I believe he kept a bag packed.

He had been an important man in the theatre and at one time a scriptwriter for British Columbia. He was one of the most remarkable men I have ever met and one of the bravest.

I made this broadcast live from Bristol.

Pam took the children to Bristol Zoo

then they listened on the car radio just outside the studios. For some reason Rolfe Whiteman decided to join in my broadcast, interjecting ums and ahs. I don't think it helped.

There was one unfortunate aspect of this particular piece, which appeared in the *Radio Times*. The broadcast was advertised as 'The Available Gentleman', and underneath it was written, 'A West Country doctor talks about his relationship with the man upstairs' — it took me some time to live that down.

Gradually I got to do more and more on *Woman's Hour*, mainly on medical topics. The awful thing was that I got on to radio programmes, not because I was brilliant or because I had anything wonderful to say, but because I was simple and said things in a straightforward way that people could understand. Friends would say to me, 'What a marvellous broadcasting technique you have,' not realising that I hadn't any technique at all; it was just me being me. I was in demand because I was safe and simple — what an achievement.

I did, amongst other programmes, some *Tuesday Calls*. These were live 'phone-ins from nine to ten in the morning. My first was with a lovely lady who did the morning exercises, Eileen Fowler, an expert on health and physical fitness. I'd written a book on backache, she'd spotted it and asked for me, thinking that I might be an authority on her subject.

Eileen Fowler's programme was very popular; when I met her she was in her seventies and looked about forty five.

I was fat and unfit at the time and during the course of the 'phone-in suggested to everybody that they went out and bought bicycles — this was probably as good a way of keeping fit as any.

My words of advice were heeded by many people, including some of my neighbours, who went out and bought bikes. Then someone put two and two together (I usually hid under some pseudonym for broadcasting) and realised that the fat slob of a man across the road had said 'Get on your bike'. This expression was subsequently picked up by some minor politician a good twenty years later, which showed how much ahead of my time I was!

I liked going up to the BBC to broadcast, and the *Woman's Hour* people were extremely nice to work with. During the time I was with them the general nature of the programmes changed and reading from scripts was abandoned in favour of not having scripts at all. This suited me much better as, unless you are an actor, it is very difficult to insert the right inflections in the right places, whereas if you just speak your own words in your own voice in your own way, it's much more convincing and, of course, it's you.

Of all the broadcasts that I did over many years — and in some of them I was trying to get deep messages across — the only complimentary remarks that I ever got from people who knew me who'd heard my broadcasts were on the following lines: 'Bob [or Doctor — depending on how well they knew me], we heard your broadcast the other day. It was marvellous. It sounded exactly like you. It could have been you standing in my kitchen [or dining room, or whatever].' They never made any comment on the content of the broadcast, just that it sounded exactly like me. How surprising. It was *me* — no wonder it sounded like me.

What they were saying wasn't quite as bad as it sounds.

Sound recording cannot reproduce the whole range of your voice, and it either flatters or distorts it. I was lucky. The radio flattered my voice and television made me look much more positive, whereas I knew a most accomplished speaker, a very distinguished lady with a very nice voice, who on the radio sounded like Mickey Mouse.

So perhaps all my friends and patients could be excused for complimenting me in the way they did.

The most stressful broadcasts of all were the *Tuesday Call* 'phone-ins. I think they were made unnecessarily alarming.

The usual set-up was to have a couple of charming, beautiful, calm ladies, like Judith Chalmers or Sue McGregor, sitting on one side of a table, plus one or two guests (to answer the questions), and a secretary at the end of the table. Outside, through a window, sat various producers, and behind them a bank of girls with telephones and then behind them a whole bank of other visitors, perhaps thirty Japanese guests touring the BBC. No wonder it could become quite stressful.

I remember once recognising one of the callers as someone who'd been at the Writers' Summer School with me in Derbyshire. It was on the tip of my tongue to say 'Hello, Jack. I hope you enjoyed last year at the Writers' Summer School. See you next year,' when it dawned on me that perhaps Jack wasn't supposed to be at the school — he might have told his wife a different story — and that would have been very much disapproved of by the BBC.

The most harrowing *Tuesday Call* I ever did was with Gill Parker, a lovely lady who was a general practitioner and the wife of the then head of British Rail. There was a rehearsal the night before, during which a lot of wine was splashed about. Afterwards I went out with some medical friends and a lot more wine was splashed about. I eventually went to bed with a headache, and couldn't settle. I was staying in a hotel in London's Half Moon Street and there seemed to be traffic going all night — it was very noisy. When I arrived at the studio in the morning, not only was I lacking in sleep, but I had an awful headache and I was also wearing, for the first time, a new pair of bi-focal glasses. Every time I looked up I felt giddy.

I sat in my chair and, glancing at the clock, realised that I had an hour's live spontaneous broadcast ahead of me. On this particular morning the subject matter was general medical questions and Gill Parker and I had to stretch ourselves to the limit to get through it.

The hour seemed like an eternity and I literally sweated it out, my head thumping. Inwardly I was swearing never to touch a drop of wine again when a question came through: 'My husband is an alcoholic. What does Doctor Clifford recommend?' I turned appealingly to Gill Parker. Bless her, she took the question in her stride and gave a very good answer — I wasn't up to it that morning.

As I started to write books I began to appear on other programmes.

I was interviewed by Esther Rantzen on *Start the Week*, chaired by the delightful Richard Baker, with Fritz Spiegel and Moira Lister (who was absolutely gorgeous) on my right to be interviewed by Kenneth Robinson; Lance Percival strummed a guitar in the background.

I was being interviewed by Esther on a funny book called *The Medical Handbook to End All Medical Handbooks*.

We were sitting quietly in a circle round a table when suddenly Kenneth Robinson got up and attacked Moira Lister rudely about a play she was in at Wimbledon. It was unbelievably embarrassing and quite uncalled for.

All the members at the table later wrote to Moira Lister saying how sorry they were, the whole attack being in the worst possible taste.

I don't know what it's called — provocative broadcasting or something — but I found it both extremely unpleasant and unjustified.

The same book got me on to *Stop the*

Week with Robert Robinson, whose other guests were Richard Gordon, Edward Du Bono, Benny Green and the literary editor of the *Manchester Guardian*.

Having two funny doctors on the same programme, I thought medical humour would be a main feature, but it wasn't. We were questioned about doctors' pay, which we knew nothing about.

We also had to give in-depth reports on a new book on adolescence by Doctor Spock. I thought it was very good and had a lot to offer, but my fellow guests were pretty noncommittal, or even damning. I felt that these were harsh judgements for them to make.

Whenever a book of my own was published and I was being interviewed on radio or television it was always fun.

I didn't have to make any preparations. Usually the interviewers have appeared interested and over the years I've been on various radio stations all over the country: the BBC's *Today, Late Night Extra*, as well as *Woman's Hour* programmes, *Home This Afternoon*, the London Broadcasting Company, Radio London, Radio 210, Radio Bristol, Radio Wiltshire,

Radio Sussex, Radio Oxford — all tremendous fun.

On the whole I found that the radio programmes were often more professional than their television counterparts.

I remember doing one 'phone-in, I think it was on first aid, for Radio London. Instead of involving masses of people, like they did on the BBC's *Tuesday Call*, an interviewer, one man on the telephone and a television monitor were all that were needed and it seemed to work more smoothly.

I literally drifted into television. I'd done a couple of things for the *Today* programme, one in answer to a fiery letter I'd written about the treatment of doctors. I had to debate the issue with a trades unionist, Lord Cooper, under the chairmanship of Kenneth Allsop. Lord Cooper and I were supposed to be on opposite sides but, in the end, we ganged up on Kenneth Allsop and I think we won.

Then one afternoon in the surgery, a panic 'phone call. Could I go up to London? It was the tenth anniversary of the National Health Service. The BBC had been looking through their files and I was about the only person who'd ever said anything nice about the National Health Service. They were interviewing the Minister of Health and wanted some doctors to say some encouraging things about it. I said I couldn't go because there was a rail strike on and I wouldn't be able to get there. The BBC suggested I caught a plane.

I rang the airports. There were no planes going to London.

After exploring every conventional avenue, my receptionist, Pam Law, said, 'You know, my husband drives to London very quickly; he'll run you up in a couple of hours.'

It was in the middle of the holiday season so I had my doubts.

Bill Law and I set off at speed, haring in and out of the traffic, overtaking everything. Everybody was tooting at us, some actually trying to run us into the hedge.

We got as far as Shaftesbury, but were so behind time I rang the BBC and told them we couldn't make it.

'Keep going,' they said. 'We'll send a

BBC car to meet you at Ruislip.'

We eventually made Ruislip and found the car. I wasn't going to miss the broadcast as I thought; the programme was an hour later than they told me.

We tore up to the BBC in the taxi, the producer met me in the foyer and said, 'I'll brief you in the lift going up. The Minister of Health is there with a few doctors. There'll be a film, then you will be questioned and you will be able to question the Minister.'

I felt like a real celebrity. I went into the studio. There were ten doctors sitting in a row. I did wonder how much time we were going to have to speak to the Minister of Health.

The programme began with a ten-minute film on the start of the National Health Service and then Michael Barratt started asking the doctors some questions. He turned to me and said, 'In what way has the new ancillary help facility of nurses in general practice helped you?'

I said, 'Our nurses syringe ears and bandage varicose veins.'

I wasn't asked any other questions.

I didn't have to say another word.

Bill Law drove me back to Tadchester at a somewhat slower pace, finally arriving at six in the morning.

My real television career started when I was interviewed by Westward Television about my first book, *The Hairy Man's Guide to First Aid*, which I wrote under the pseudonym of Doctor Pheasant.

They had a great laugh in the studio; people dressed up in rugby clothes threw water over each other, struggled to give mouth-to-mouth resuscitation — it was great fun.

After the programme I was asked if I would become the programme's resident doctor, i.e. appear about once a month and put into simple language various medical problems that might arise.

They were a very nice young team at Westward.

The chief presenter, Kenneth McCleod, was a most accomplished actor and broadcaster.

Amongst the rest of the team was Angela Rippon, as lovely a young girl as she is now a mature woman and a first-class interviewer. At one time she had her own woman's programme and I appeared on it to talk about a book I had written called *How to Put on Weight*.

This particular book had more media coverage than any other I've ever produced — it also sold less. It was good to talk about, but not to buy. Anglia Television also interviewed me about this book, but it was through a link-up from a London studio and I had to speak into a monitor. It was quite disconcerting — every time I answered a question from the interviewer my own face came up on the monitor and I had to speak to myself.

At Westward Television I made perhaps the worst six first-aid films of all time. I was asked if I could do it, foolishly agreed and suddenly realised I had to script and present the series.

I had no idea how to go about it. We used to film it in the lunchtimes, to the disgust of all the various studio workers, i.e. lighting men, scene shifters, etc. I remember we spent a long session showing how to cope with a cut finger, which involved holding the finger under a tap, putting some disinfectant on it, then putting on some Elastoplast tape. When we came to look at it afterwards, it was thought to be so bad we had to do it again.

Harlech Television also interviewed me on the *How to Put on Weight* book, and afterwards I was asked to become the resident doctor on their *Women Only* programme, where a very young Jan Leeming was the presenter. This was a splendid show and years later when Jan Leeming became nationally famous as a newsreader, I always thought that so much of her talent was wasted. She was one of the best and most professional programme presenters that I've ever come across.

I did some interviewing on the *Women Only* programme for Harlech. I first interviewed a doctor's wife on her book about the National Health Service.

I made the mistake of giving away all my most penetrating questions when I was discussing the book with the author prior to the broadcast. Of course, when the broadcast time came round she had thought out new answers to my questions and I was the one to be non-plussed. I had to put it all down to experience.

I was next to interview the great Claire

Rayner about her second novel, *A Time to Heal*.

It was arranged that I would go up to Paddington to meet her, then we were to travel down to Bristol together and discuss her novel over breakfast.

Claire is a marvellous person, has more energy than three people put together, and, I believe, employs six secretaries. She is a really lovely genuine lady, in the fullest sense of the word. This has been recently confirmed in a survey to find the best-liked woman in the country. She came second to Felicity Kendall.

Claire is also one of the great talkers of the world, on a par with Maeve Binchey. If ever I was asked to form a government, I would appoint Claire as prime minister and Maeve as foreign secretary, they would sweep everything before them, nobody would get a chance to get a word in edgeways; Margaret Thatcher is not in their league. I, of course, would be in charge of the Treasury.

Claire and I talked non-stop all the way to Bristol. She told me she wanted to write an operetta, and an on-going saga of novels following a family over a period of 150 years. It all sounded like pie in the sky, but she was true to her word, she produced a twelve-book bestselling series, as well as continuing with her agony aunt column, newspaper and magazine articles and radio and television. I last saw her at a publishing party in March, 1988. She looked just as fit and bouncing with energy as she had done when I had interviewed her back in 1972.

Because we were talking so much, we hardly touched our breakfast. As the train pulled into Bristol, we realised we hadn't actually got round to discussing her novel, which had been the object of the exercise.

It didn't matter. Claire is a very easy person to interview. I hailed her as the new H.G. Wells. *A Time to Heal* was about a cancer cure, and Claire had predicted all sorts of things like test-tube babies, long before they were implemented.

Some months later we were again on Harlech Television together. I don't know what Claire's contribution was, but mine was to talk about what a doctor carries in his bag, and for the only time on TV I had my medical case with me.

Claire and I travelled back by rail together and sat in the restaurant car at the back of the train.

Out in the wilds of the country the train made an unscheduled stop. A guard came along to explain that a man had been hit on the line.

I said, 'Well, I'm a doctor, and this lady is a nurse. Can we be of any assistance?'

'I don't know the exact position,' said the guard, 'but if you could make your way to the front of the train, I'm sure they would be extremely grateful.'

I grabbed my medical case, and Claire and I ran the whole length of the train, with me shouting 'I'm a doctor!' and Claire shouting, 'I'm a nurse!', whenever someone impeded our progress.

It seemed like miles before we reached the front of the train. We were helped down the steep drop to the ground, and led round to the front of the engine where two labourers were shovelling the remains of what had been a man on to a wheelbarrow. We trudged our way slowly back to the restaurant car, answering

'Everything is under control,' to anyone who asked. I never learnt who the poor fellow was or whether it was an accident or suicide; I don't think that Claire or I will ever forget it.

There is a public side to Claire, which is seen to engage in a prodigious amount of work. I also know that there is a private one that is just as busy, as there have been occasions when she has rung me about some medical aspect of a problem she is dealing with personally. She is a truly marvellous human being. I am unable to make the 'Wellsian' predictions that Claire makes, but I would very much like to predict that one day she will be honoured by being made a Dame. If she isn't, then she should be.

I enjoyed both radio and television, although I was very much on the periphery. I was never particularly well known as a broadcaster, but I did relish the atmosphere of the studio and loved meeting the people taking part in programmes, particularly in Harlech Television's *Women Only* programme, which always had a host of interesting celebrities.

It was a tremendous experience and so different from my world of medicine that it was a great help in maintaining my own equilibrium with all the problems and tragedies that I had to deal with in my daily round. It gave me a foothold in another camp and although ninety-five per cent of my time was spent in medicine, meeting all these people in a different world was my relaxation and a great stabiliser.

My last television appearance was in series called *Believe it or not*. It was chaired by Paul Heiney, Andy Price and a lovely girl from the TV series *Crossroads*. The item I was involved in was to feature in a pilot programme and, if all went well, in the first programme. There were to be six programmes and six components of each.

My particular spot related to Culpeper's *London Dispensatory* of the seventeenth century. This was a famous book detailing the pharmaceutical preparations that were used in those days, like dead bodies, stag's pizzel and elf hearts, and we were looking to see how many of them were still being used today.

Old-fashioned remedies had become topical, and leeches, for example, were once more proving useful in medicine, particularly in eye surgery.

We had a good pilot programme and it was decided to go ahead with the series.

In the first episode, where I did my piece about how medical preparations came and went over the years, Andy Price went into the audience and talked to some of the studio guests on camera.

Trevor and a friend were my guests and they were both interviewed. How nice, I thought, that we should both be on the same television programme together.

However, it was not to be. Somewhere along the line (and it was blamed on the Director General of the BBC) it was thought that the six programmes weren't up to scratch. They scrambled the six programmes they'd made, taking out the best items to make just three programmes.

I watched the programme when it

was eventually broadcast. They didn't interfere with my piece but they chopped and changed the others around so much it became very confusing. One minute, for example, you'd see Paul Heiney in a green jersey, and the next minute he'd be in a yellow one, as they jumped from one episode to another.

I thought the programme I was in was excellent and the people I worked with were all terribly nice. They were all very upset about it being broken up. Knowing there was little chance of my appearing on television again, and having little to lose, I wrote a long letter to the supposed villain of the piece, Derek Hart, who was the then Director General of the BBC.

I received a charming reply, thanking me for my letter, saying he would find out who had cancelled the programme and ask them to write to me and explain why it had been edited as it had. He would also ask the said producer/director to send him a copy of the letter. So the Director General wasn't the culprit, it was somebody else; whoever it was, I would certainly never be his favourite person.

I received an explanatory letter in due course, and an exceedingly long one at that (remember, this man had to send a copy to the Director General).

He started by saying that if only the contents of the programme had been up to the standard of my contribution, of course, they would have had no trouble. I took this with the great pinch of salt with which it was intended. Unfortunately, he said, most of the other items fell far beneath the standard of my performance.

To me it seemed that he had dodged the responsibility for reducing the programme and passed the buck, and suddenly the buck had come back to him. I winced as I read his letter; I knew that somewhere I had made a deadly enemy. I felt pretty certain that nobody would ever invite me to appear on a BBC television programme again, and I was absolutely right. I was never asked and never appeared again.

10

Singing for Supper

ALTHOUGH I now live in the south midlands and have written mainly about the west of England, the only real literary occasions I have been invited to speak at are in the north of England. *The Yorkshire Ridings' Magazine* were very kind to me, as were the *Lancashire Magazine*, and I did a number of speaking engagements for them at dinners and lunches. They usually coincided with the publication of a new book and involved signing sessions after the meal.

My first actual literary dinner was for the *Yorkshire Ridings' Magazine* in Bradford, and was shared with a delightful policeman author called Peter Walker. I had become pretty sure of myself as a speaker, in fact, a bit too sure. A few weeks before the Bradford dinner I'd gone back to the

Writers' Summer School at Swanwick in Derbyshire, as one of the celebrity speakers, some twenty years after having first gone there as a 'new boy' without having anything published or broadcast.

We had a good dinner in Bradford, with perhaps a couple of hundred people in attendance. The publisher's representative had been brought back from holiday because of the dinner and I looked forward to a most enjoyable evening, not least because of hearing myself speak.

We had our meal then Peter spoke. He turned out to be a first-class speaker. At literary lunches and dinners, particularly, it's very difficult to follow someone who speaks well, especially if they've been amusing. If you've wined and dined well, and been amused and entertained, you often feel ready to go home after a good speaker.

My turn came. I got up full of confidence but made the great mistake of reading something that I thought was funny. Being a bad reader of scripts my talk didn't go down well at all. If only Peter Walker hadn't been quite so good

I might have held the attention of the audience a bit better.

I rate my talks or speeches as wins, loses or draws, and this was definitely a loss.

At the end of the dinner we had to leave the dining room to go to a second room. I was escorted by this poor rep who had foreshortened his holiday, and there, on a table, were my books for sale, dozens of them in rows.

I got out my pen, ready to sign, but this wasn't to be my evening: A good crowd collected around Peter Walker, and, not only did nobody buy my book, but also nobody even spoke to me, except, just as the evening was drawing to a close, a man who walked up and said how much he loved books and that most of his friends were doctors.

I joined the queue at Peter's table and bought one of his books. Bless him, he repaid the compliment and bought one of mine. I hated to think what the publisher's rep must have thought about his ruined holiday.

We were being put up by the *Yorkshire Ridings' Magazine* at the Olde Silent Inn at Stanbury, on the moors near Howarth, a lovely old place. I went back in despair; I felt I'd let them down. 'Don't worry,' said Winston, managing director of the magazine, 'you've got to be professional about these things. You win some, you lose some — it may be quite different tomorrow.' His words of comfort were endorsed by Joan Laprell, the features editor, both lovely people who became great friends over the years.

But I had a restless night, picking over my speech. Winston had tactfully said, and he was quite right, that reading something was perhaps not the best thing.

I knew that I had to face an audience at Halifax at a function the next day.

Winston was right — I had a completely different reception at Halifax. The speech went over well, I didn't bore them to tears by reading something, and when it came to the book-signing session, there was a whole queue of people buying books, as well as a whole lot more coming up to talk about books and writing. A most delightful occasion, and my confidence was restored.

My next literary occasion for this magazine was a great honour. It was during the Barnsley Book Week, and apparently more people in Barnsley take out library books than in anywhere else in the world. There was to be a dinner in the evening and a lunch the following day at the same venue. I was in most distinguished company here and we were billed as bestselling authors, which I wasn't — I considered myself as a sort of aperitif before the main course.

At the literary dinner in the evening the other two speakers were the marvellous James Herriot and the incredible Jeffrey Archer, and I certainly wasn't in their league but this was part of the fun I got out of writing.

At lunch the following day Jeffrey Archer was again one of the speakers and the other was a much underestimated writer, and a man who, over the years, became a great friend. Sadly he was taken terminally ill just a couple of days before he was due to spend a weekend with us at Wallingford and he was so looking forward to a trip on the boat. He was an author who had really reached a peak with one of his first novels, *Room at the Top* — of course, I'm referring to John Braine. He told me that just after *Room at the Top* was published he was approached by both the Conservative and Labour parties to stand as a candidate. He wisely refused both offers. John was a truly professional author, a disciplined writer whose manuscripts always arrived on time.

It was not always easy to get to know the real John under that rather bluff, almost aggressive, exterior, but he was a very kindly learned man and was full of commonsense.

Jeffrey Archer was a brilliant speaker. Fortunately I didn't have to follow him because he insisted on speaking last. At the luncheon at Barnsley this did not work to my advantage. I had been a Bevin Boy just at the end of the War, coal-mining in South Yorkshire. My colliery had not been too far away from Barnsley and I'd had an uncle in Maltby whom I often visited at weekends when I was there.

He died some years ago but I was very fond of my Uncle George and as I got up to speak, Uncle George and Maltby were very much in my mind because I was going to mention him fairly early on.

I started my speech by saying, 'This is my first visit to Maltby,' and had only completed a few sentences when I realised that, of course, this was my first visit to Barnsley not Maltby and I had to start again. I don't know what Jeffrey had prepared to say prior to my speech, but he devoted most of his allotted ten minutes to saying how confused he was because he thought he'd come to Barnsley and now he found he was in Maltby. He'd have to sack his agent, and where was Maltby anyway? I decided definitely not to vote for him at the next election.

Going to dinners and lunches up north allowed me to revisit areas that I'd known in the past, mainly from just at the end of the War and, of course, I am a Yorkshireman by birth. It was amazing how things had changed. In 1946 there seemed to be smoke and slag-heaps in evidence from Watford onwards, but now, as you go north, it is difficult to spot a mine or black smoke anywhere.

John Braine and I travelled to Preston to do a lunch and a dinner there for the *Lancashire Magazine* and I was amazed how clean and neat everything was. The girls from the magazine took me for a ride in the country in the morning before the luncheon, and I thought that the supposedly industrial north was more countrified and generally in better order than the south. The streets seemed to be cleaner, with no litter about, and overall a better sense of order prevailed. It was a real pleasure.

Another time, I did a literary lunch and dinner in Keighley with the marvellous Maeve Binchey who, as well as being one of our best contemporary novelists, is without any doubt the best after-dinner speaker I have heard. She is an absolute riot.

Before the dinner Maeve asked very sweetly, would I mind if she spoke first as she was a bit nervous?

I would have much preferred speaking first but, being the gentleman I am, I agreed. Maeve was brilliant and I had the most difficult time following her. I made my talk short and sweet; I could have listened to her all night.

The next day we were to attend a luncheon and book-signing session at Nostell Priory, a magnificent old country house. This time I made sure that my short and sweet contribution was delivered before Maeve brought the house down. I would love to be able to write her after-dinner stories, but I'm sure that one day we will see them all in print.

I managed to persuade Maeve and her husband Gordon, and John Braine and Janet Barber, to come down to Plymouth for the West of England Writers' Congress (of which I was vice-chairman), where I had the greatest pleasure of all, being able to sit back and listen to them without having to contribute myself.

It seemed that I was doomed to literary lunches only in the north of England. There was a one-off half way down, a literary lunch at Ross-on-Wye where the other authors were the lovely Dulcie Gray, a most prolific and excellent novelist, Michael Dennison and Peter York, who co-wrote the extremely successful *Sloane Rangers' Handbook*.

My old friend Robin Treaton came down from Birmingham as my guest at this luncheon. To my surprise, I sold a great number of books — apparently Robin had practically bludgeoned people into buying them. I thought I'd have to take him with me to every literary occasion.

I once was called upon to give a lecture, not a literary one, in my own home town.

Every year the good vicar of Wallingford, namely the Reverend Good, organises five Lent lectures and he invites people from different walks of life to speak in the lovely old town hall. The speakers are not necessarily religious people, more a cross-section of society. There's usually a central theme each year which relates to Christianity or the Church. The year before my lecture the theme had been ethics, and we went to hear Richard Ingrams speak on the ethics of journalism. He has a bookshop in Wallingford and although he's not the person who immediately springs to mind when this subject is under discussion, he gave a first-class talk. During his lecture

I sat next to a lady who had brought her very young baby with her and, just as Richard Ingrams started to talk, it started to cry. Without a moment's hesitation, she pulled up her jumper exposing a bare bosom, stuck her baby on it and it suckled happily through the lecture, and why not? It would be interesting to know if in twenty years' time the baby becomes a gifted journalist.

In my year the theme of the lectures was the media. I had to talk on the media, medicine and the Church. I felt a bit out of my depth. Other speakers included Michael Grade's deputy talking about television and the Church; somebody else spoke on communications and the Church. I worked harder at this lecture than I have done for any other and by my reckoning would have rated it a draw.

Having resigned myself to always speaking in the north of England, out of the blue the London Street Bookshop at Reading asked me to speak at the civic centre to the UK Federation of Business and Professional Women. This was only sixteen miles from home and I thought a step in the right direction.

I do not know Reading very well, and do not enjoy driving into it. I set off on the Oxford – Reading road, which is a beautiful undulating run with wide expanses of fields and woods, coming into Reading over Caversham Bridge. This was the easy bit. Then I plunged into the subterranean maze that leads to the Hexagon, the civic centre and the Butts shopping centre. I thought that speaking at the civic centre might give me privileged parking, so warily picked my way through underground passages to a place where an official was putting some bollards down and where a notice proclaimed 'Civic centre car park'.

I explained to him that I was speaking at the civic centre but, instead of welcoming me, he directed me towards the Butts multi-storey car park, which caters for the big shopping centre. There was a long, winding ascending ramp that I felt had a sinister atmosphere about it. I went through the bottom of the ramp, expecting an automatic ticket machine, but there was no barrier or anything.

I drove up the long ramp, parked and looked round for signs about payment.

There was none to be seen.

I came out of the first exit, went down to the civic centre and met the lady from the London Street Bookshop. I enquired as to whether the Butts car park was free at night and was assured that this was so. We went to the room in which the meeting was to be held but found it already occupied by a group of ten or so men having a meeting. On an indicator board outside, the business women's meeting was allocated to a much smaller room. As we went into our room, I wondered if someone had been switching the room markers. Not only was it quite inadequate for the numbers coming to the meeting, but also it had not been cleared up after the last occupants. There were tables arranged down the middle of the room, piled with dirty coffee cups and trays. To save time, these energetic business ladies rolled up their sleeves and cleared away the coffee cups etc., piled up the tables, and crammed in chairs to hold the anticipated numbers. Slowly the room filled up with lady accountants, nurses, bankers, solicitors, health visitors, etc.

Later than expected, the chairperson, who had been held up in a traffic jam, came into the room in a soaking wet blouse. I wondered if she'd been posing for *Playboy* pictures but she assured me she had only been drenched in wine, which I thought was better still! (Apparently it was all quite innocent — she'd been carrying some boxes of wine for the do afterwards and one of them had burst, covering her.)

It was the fulfilment of one of my ambitions: there was I, the only man in a party of forty attractive women. I only wished there was some way I could have joined their Society.

We had a good meeting and they very kindly bought lots of books; in fact, it's the only time that I've ever sold out.

When it was all over, I went up into the gloom of the Butts centre, got into my car and drove home.

Three or four days later, when we were getting the car out, Pam noticed something wrapped round my windscreen wiper. It was a note saying I'd been fined £15 for parking in the Butts car park without a ticket. I hit the roof. I sent a long letter to the chief executive of Reading Council saying how difficult it was to pay for something if there was nowhere obvious to pay.

I went on to elaborate about the room that I spoke in, saying it was the first time I'd had to clear a room of tables, cups and chairs before I spoke and I said I looked forward to his comments. To the Council's great credit and, on enquiring, I found that if I had walked further into the car park, there were big 'pay and display' signs. However, they wrote back to me with a letter of apology, waiving the fine.

My next speaking engagement after Reading was, of course, back up north again. This was to a library lecture at a literary week in Stockport. The actual venue was Cheadle Hulme Library. This was quite exciting because I'd been to Cheadle Hulme School when I was eight. I was able to go back and have a look at the house where I'd lived fifty years before, and the lady who lives there now very kindly showed me round.

I'd had to catch the only convenient non-stop train from Didcot to Stockport, which meant that Barry Richards, an old friend and the Pelham rep for the area, had to meet me at lunchtime and entertain me for the day. He offered me about six options, one of which was to go home to have a salad, which we decided to do. I thought it would put him to the least trouble. To my utter amazement he produced fifteen different types of salads, plus quiches, pates and all sorts. He kindly took me round to my old house and Cheadle Hulme School and when his wife Linda arrived home in the evening, I was offered a choice of haute cuisine dishes. Not wishing to cause them any extra work, I said I'd be very happy with an omelette, only to see the family tucking into the likes of chicken Kiev, coq au vin and poached salmon. And then when it came to a sweet, again there were about a dozen different desserts to choose from. 'So this is how publishers' reps live, is it, Barry?' I asked. But there was a secret behind it — they'd had a party the day before and some guests couldn't come so they'd had an abundance of food left over.

But I didn't let them get away with it.

From then on whenever I wrote to Barry and Linda I addressed them as Mr and Mrs Richards, Caterers.

They were a most hospitable couple: Barry not only took me sight-seeing, fed me, ferried me to the meetings and back to my hotel, but also insisted on picking me up at 8 o'clock the following morning and running me to the station.

My talk to the UK Federation of Business and Professional Women in Reading had introduced me to southern society, and we had a marvellous literary dinner at the new Ramada Hotel, Reading, where the other two speakers were Nigel Rees, who's written a huge number of books, is an expert on graffiti, a well-known radio and television personality and who has now written his first (excellent) novel, *The News Makers*. The star of the evening and a great person to meet was Willie Rushton, one of England's really true wits. It was an extremely successful evening. It was a lovely hotel and we were able to get a lot of our friends to come along and I was quite amazed at the numbers of books that were sold in one evening.

One thing leads to another. Following the Ramada I was booked to speak to a Writing for Pleasure class in Newbury, invited to give a lecture at the Reading Literary Festival in June with a repeat performance in Stockport, this time to speak to the Conservative Ladies' Supper Club. Apparently they'd only ever had one other author and that was Jeffrey Archer when he was doing pre-election literary lunches. I was glad he wasn't going to be there as I'm sure I would have started off by saying, 'This is the first time I've been to Sale' or some other place than the one I was actually in.

I think all these literary-type occasions are of great benefit to the writer, though not in commercial terms. If you add up the profit made on the books sold at any luncheon or dinner, it's unlikely that it would pay the train fare to the venue, never mind the hotel bill. The main benefit, from the author's point of view, is publicity, which is always useful and, of course, it's good for your ego.

Writing is an isolated, lonely business and being flattered by having a captive public audience to listen to you speaking about your own work is a great boost to your morale.

In recent years writers have tended to get together more. The most important gathering of budding authors is the Writers' Summer School in Derby where about four hundred writers live under the same roof for one week. There is also the West Country Writers' Association. To join this latter set you must have some connection with the West Country, or have written about the West Country and had at least a couple of hardback books published. I was their secretary for three years and remember the first conference I organised for them. We had many distinguished people, such as Henry Williamson, Kenneth Allsop, the President, Christopher Fry, and our guest of honour was Jenny Lee, then Minister for Arts. The West Country Writers' meetings were rather special in that they weren't workshops like most writing weekends. We would meet in a different West Country town each year, and the local authorities always gave us a civic reception. We had an annual general meeting and a few celebrated speakers, a

150

large luncheon and then usually theatre on the Saturday evening.

I remember the first one that I organised in Exeter. Pam and I had to escort Christopher Fry and Jenny Lee to the Northcott Theatre to see *The Tempest* performed in Edwardian dress, and afterwards the cast lined up to receive Christopher Fry and Jenny Lee as if they were royalty.

There are now writing weekends and organisations which have sprung up all over the country, mainly created by people who have been unable to get into the Derbyshire summer school, so there are alternatives if you're not one of the lucky four hundred.

One year I was a speaker and chairman of the Southern Writers' Conference at Chichester. I went up to speak at the Scarborough Writers' Weekend, travelling up on the train with the star of the weekend, Margaret Drabble, John Braine being one of the other speakers. I was a guest at the Leicester Writers' Circle, many of whom were established writers, and presented the prizes at their annual dinner. I also had a lovely weekend in the

151

Lake District with the Northern Writers, in a beautiful lakeside hotel.

It's unlikely that I would have got into print or been invited to any of these occasions unless I'd been a doctor. Everybody has a consuming interest in medicine of some sort or another, and writing is something you can pursue from your home without it interfering with your job. You don't have to move house, or change your wife, and you can have a new career and explore the world with your pen without ever leaving your front door or giving up the way you earn your daily bread.

We all need our own formula for survival and mine was to practise medicine and dabble in writing and be involved with writers.

I used to say that I was completely schizophrenic: my doctor friends thought of me as a writer and my writer friends thought of me as a doctor. But this, in fact, was quite true. Somehow, confining myself to one rôle was more than I could cope with: I had to give an excuse for any inadequacies I might present in either rôle.

The main benefit of my writing was not financial — this was small — it was the fact that it helped me take a more balanced view of life. Wordsworth said, 'A poet's job is to describe people's experiences,' and of course, so is a writer's. Being a medical writer I was able, through my own experiences and those of the people I dealt with, to give comfort to others having to face similar situations. So, through my writing I was also practising medicine.

I will never, ever consider that I am a real writer. Real writers are creative people who explore new barriers. I'm just somebody who records day-to-day events, and as a doctor I have had privileged access to other people's lives. I consider myself fortunate to have had a few books published.

11

It's Quicker by Tube

ALTHOUGH now officially retired from active medicine, I still do a lot of counselling on the telephone. Barely a day goes by without a former patient ringing me to chat about his or her particular ailments. I try to keep in touch by reading medical journals, noting all the incredible strides that medicine is making — unbelievable brain transplants, laser surgery, etc.

Amazing things were beginning to happen in the few years before I retired, particularly in the field of midwifery.

I experienced for the first time the techniques involved in test-tube babies and other new procedures which gave childless couples the opportunity of having a family that they otherwise wouldn't have had. This remarkable achievement usually solved all sorts of other problems for the couples involved, as was illustrated all too well in the case of Steven and Sonia Martin.

Steven and Sonia were favourite patients of mine. I had known them literally since birth, having attended both their arrivals as home confinements, back in the days when home was the usual place to be born. After Sonia's birth the family sent me a dozen bottles of champagne. As a result of all this I was an honoured guest at their wedding, sitting at the top table.

It was totally undeserved, as my only contribution to Sonia's arrival in the world was to sit drinking a cup of tea while our then midwife, the admirable Nurse Plank, did all the hard work.

Much of the credit one receives in general practice is not merited, as are the complaints but, as an elderly physician from Winchcombe once observed, we tend to get more than our fair share of praise.

Sonia and Steven were a very good-looking couple, and played a lively part in the young people's activities in the town.

Steven was captain of the Tadchester Rugby Club as well as being chairman of the Round Table. Sonia played hockey for Tadchester Ladies and was a busy member of the Inner Circle. Both played tennis, swam, surfed, sailed and took part in most physical activities that were going on.

They were quite delightful, had been a 'pair' since leaving school, and had been regular mates (probably in the full sense of the word) for seven years until their marriage.

There was little doubt that their marriage was going to be a success. Steven was an accountant; Sonia worked in a bank. They had a nice house, no financial worries and were quite the leaders of young Tadchester society.

They had been married about three years when I first began to notice something was amiss. They began to come into the surgery from time to time, separately, complaining of minor problems such as headaches, indigestion, insomnia. When we met socially, they seemed to have lost their sparkle; not that anyone could go on sparkling forever, but I couldn't help sensing that something was really wrong.

They began to visit me more frequently. Sonia began to exhibit the signs of an acute depression; Steven, also on the depressive side, began to drop hints that there were problems with the physical side of their marriage, in particular that the marital act was becoming more difficult for him. The collective signs and symptoms were suggestive of a third party mucking up their marriage. This I doubted; I would have known about it beforehand — in Tadchester you couldn't get away with anything; patients would even tell me if they saw Pam going into a bank.

Sonia's depression became progressively worse, and I couldn't get to the root of the problem. It was time for some positive action: I sent them a note saying I would like to see them together at the surgery.

After making and cancelling a couple of appointments they eventually came, puzzled about why I had sent for them, sitting sullenly in front of my desk with no sign of the togetherness that had been the hallmark of their relationship over a decade.

'Sonia and Steven,' I said, 'I've known you both now since the day you were born; you are more than just patients, and I'm worried about you both. Something is wrong and I don't know what it is. Won't you tell me and see if I can help?'

At this Sonia burst into tears. 'You tell him, Steven,' she sobbed — and then it all came out. All their friends had children, and although they had tried continually since they were first married they had not managed to conceive. This had become such an issue between them that Steven was now barely potent. Each thought it must be the other's fault.

'You silly pair,' I said. 'Why on earth didn't you come and see me before? This is a very common problem and there are all sorts of things we can do about it. From now on you tackle this problem with me.'

Facing the problem with me made a great difference to them. I gave both of them a general examination, could find nothing amiss, and arranged for them to be investigated at an infertility clinic.

Rarely was this unsuccessful — but what was surprising was the number of patients who became pregnant before ever reaching the clinic. It was as if just facing up to the issue gave them some sort of release that made conception possible.

Unfortunately with Steven and Sonia this was not the case. Over the next three years they underwent every infertility test known to the medical profession. There were sperm counts, inspection of fallopian tubes, infertility drugs, monitoring of vaginal temperatures, all to no avail. All the tests were encouraging but, in spite of the various drugs given to Sonia, they still didn't conceive. It was no comfort to them that I was able to tell them truthfully that, even in these circumstances, I had patients who had still gone on to conceive.

After three years of hoping, the couple were back in the depths of despair. Sonia was acutely depressed and Steven was barely potent again.

One evening they came to see me together, with very determined looks in their faces. Steven, who had obviously been nominated spokesman, took some time to get to the point. 'We would like a test tube . . . I mean a test-tube baby,' he said. 'Whatever it costs.' They sat holding hands, looking defiantly at me.

'In your circumstances,' I said, 'this is a perfectly sensible sort of action. I have no experience of the procedure, but I will try and find something out as soon as possible.'

Sonia came round the desk and hugged me, tears streaming down her face and sobbing, 'Oh, thank you, Doctor Bob, for being so understanding!'

At the time, this procedure was not available under the National Health Service and it took a while to find out who to send them to. Eventually everything was organised and they went up to a clinic near London.

It was found that there was no reason why they should not have a baby by this method, and although they were unsuccessful at their first attempt, Sonia's second admission produced results. She conceived twins, and nine months later gave birth to two healthy boys in a London hospital.

Once her pregnancy had been confirmed, Sonia asked if there was any chance of my keeping up the family tradition and delivering her offspring at home. I now delivered only about one baby a year, so it was a definite no. This was science-fiction medicine; hospital, and a special unit at that, was the only place for her.

The twins were the answer to Steven's and Sonia's problems. Depression and impotence disappeared, and the pair returned to being the happy young couple they used to be.

Medicine has made some great advances, test-tube babies being one of the more spectacular ones. There are still some problems to sort out in this field, like what to do with spare embryos and the ethics of research on embryos. There is also the frightening thought that you could freeze an embryo in liquid nitrogen in 1988 and, as far as one knows, keep it indefinitely . . .

But, these are problems for someone else — the Church, the state, the medical profession, who knows?

From my point of view it had been the means of restoring to good health a lovely young couple, with the added bonus of two strapping boys becoming part of a loving, caring household.

12

How to Get a Book Published

WHEN I was in general practice, I had found the pressures difficult to cope with. My main energies were taken up accepting the responsibilities that went with the job.

Sometimes you had to act on impulse and have faith in your own judgement. You couldn't always be right; you could only try your best and be as careful and conscientious as possible.

You also, however difficult, had to come to terms with the fact that you could not be all things to all men.

I had been lucky that the Tadchester hospital consultants were always ready to give advice and were willing to see patients in their own homes. We had a good relationship with the main hospital ten miles away, where there were full-time specialists and where we sent our more serious cases. As the local hospital

163

began to reduce its services, more and more of our cases went to the main hospital. I hated to admit it but, in some ways, it was a relief.

Before, the vast majority of cases went into the local cottage hospital where we looked after them ourselves; now, once you knew a case was safely in an ambulance, it was somebody else's responsibility, the patient was going to somebody who was better equipped, somewhere where there was a bigger team, somewhere where there were people with more specialised knowledge than we had.

In spite of all the stresses and strains that I had in general practice, including the awful trauma of a child dying while I was anaesthetising him, and deaths in the young and people whom I had known well, the area that I had not thought would be a main area of pressure, particularly never of strain, was my hobby of writing.

It had long been my ambition to write humorous books about medicine: one, because I enjoyed writing; two, because I think that writing is an important medium of communication.

It was interesting to hear from the editor of one woman's magazine to which I contributed, that the commonest single question she was asked for advice about by parents was masturbation in small children. I had never ever been consulted by a parent about this.

People liked the anonymity of confiding in someone they didn't know.

I realised that simple medical stories could possibly be of great comfort to people who were having frightening experiences. They would see that other people had these experiences, survived them, and that they weren't all that frightening after all.

I wrote a series of articles based on this theme, called *Our Village*, for one of the 'give-away' medical magazines, and when I had done a good number, enough to form a nucleus of a book with continuity of characters, I started to submit them to newspapers, thinking they might be serialised.

I tried every national daily and every national Sunday at least twice, without any result.

Then I sent them to streams of publishers, always with a negative reply.

I was also writing a number of lay medical articles and had been commissioned by a publisher to write a book on how to put on weight. One of my patients had said that he hadn't read it but kept a copy in the back of his car for a month and found that he had put on three pounds.

The publisher thought that in every office there was a thin girl who desperately wanted to wear a bikini, or a sleeveless sweater but was too bony to risk it.

It was good media material; however, hardly anybody bought the book but it did result in a leading British magazine asking me to write an article on the subject.

I managed to arrange a lunch with the deputy editor of the magazine. My article was misprinted but that didn't really matter very much as during the luncheon this very powerful deputy editor looked at me and said, 'Can you write anecdotal humorous medicine?'

'I think so,' I said, my ears pricking at the idea.

'Right,' he said. 'Go and write me three thousand words and I'll pay you a hundred pounds for the option of buying it.'

I, of course, already had thirty or forty thousand words written, so I sent him a sample three days later.

He was on the 'phone straightaway. 'This is marvellous stuff,' he said. 'Now write me thirty thousand words.'

I polished up the material I had already written, and sent it to him.

I was immediately summoned to lunch in the executive suite of this massive publishing house.

Coincidentally I had a friend in publishing who had edited all the other work I had done before. This was mainly on medical matters. He was moving to a general publishing house and said he would be happy to publish a book of my stories. It seemed as if all my dreams were coming true at once.

I managed to arrange for him to attend lunches with the deputy editor and features editor of this great magazine.

It was quite frightening. The building was huge. You could have got virtually the whole of my West Country town inside it.

This magazine, which was world famous, had a floor of its own and before one of the eventual five lunches that we had with these two very senior people, I was taken round the whole of the office and introduced as their new, bestselling author.

They were delighted with the stuff that I had provided.

Not only were they going to publish it, but were also going to use it as the basis of their new-year television advertising as a balance to some articles they had done about a politician who had disgraced himself.

I thought I was going to become rich and famous.

I went to London for the final lunch, after which we were to sign the contracts. Also joining us for lunch was a delightful chap from a national daily, who was to do the actual serialisation.

I came bounding in, smiling, to meet frosty faces that remained so over lunch.

I was attacked by the deputy editor. Lord knows why.

Whether he had over-reached himself in some way or not I don't know, but I had changed in one week from being the best thing since sliced bread, to being an awful writer.

If only I could write like I talked, he said.

The only chance that the book might be serialised would be if the journalist could make something of it, and it was pretty doubtful that he could.

There would be no contracts signed today.

With this anticipated success I had managed to persuade a literary agent to take me on to guard my interests. I 'phoned her about the whole thing. She was quite bemused.

She said, 'There's nothing we can do about it. We'll just have to wait and see.'

The nice man from the national daily came down to see me at home and agreed to serialise my anecdotal stories. A fortnight later I had a 'phone call from the deputy editor saying that the stories were absolutely terrific and we would soon have a celebration lunch. I could have kicked myself for having so little faith.

After three or four weeks, having not heard about this celebration lunch, I rang the deputy editor to say that I felt this celebration lunch ought to be on me; I had already had five lunches on them.

He, rather cautiously, replied in a tone that gave rise to all sorts of uncertainties. He would prefer to get in touch with me, he said.

He did get in touch with me a week later. I had a letter saying they had decided not to do the serialisation of my work.

It was quite beyond my comprehension. I poured out my woes to my editor friend.

'Don't worry,' he said, 'we've still got the book to look forward to and that's coming on nicely.'

One month later the famous magazine sent a secretary in a taxi round to his publishing house saying that they wanted a copy of the manuscript of the book immediately.

They had decided to serialise it in their magazine after all, at the end of the next month.

A copy of what we had done so far was hastily assembled, bundled into the taxi, and we were smiling once more. Oh, we of little faith.

A month passed and nothing happened. I asked my agent to enquire as to the fate of my serialisation (I daren't ring them up myself).

She rang me back and said, 'I'm very sorry to say that they have decided, again, not to do it after all.'

I did wonder whether magazine editors ever slept at night; I understand they have a pretty high mortality rate.

I thought it might be worth trying to have the stories serialised somewhere else. When we had got near to finishing them in book form, I sent them to one of the national Sunday papers that I had contributed to in the past but they returned them saying they were sorry, it wasn't for them.

'Never mind,' said my book editor. 'The book's going to come out. Stop worrying. It'll hold its own.'

And it did come out. It had a smashing cover, now all that it needed was people to buy it.

The new book had been out one week when my book editor rang.

'Bob,' he said. 'I have some bad news for you.'

'Come on,' I said, 'tell me the worst.'

He said, 'I'm afraid the receivers are in.'

His new publishing firm had gone bankrupt. I thought this was the end, but in the dying moments of the publishing house the publicity officer had sent some review copies out. The national Sunday paper that turned my book down for serialisation, gave the book the most marvellous review any author could wish for. It must have struck a chord in the reviewer's heart for I felt he gave it a better review than it deserved. The newspaper, now reading the review in its own columns, decided they would serialise it after all.

My agent, God bless her, as soon as she heard that the publishing house was in receivership, got in a taxi and rescued the manuscript. Within a month we had a serialisation in a national Sunday paper pending, and had sold the book to a large established publishing house who turned out to be honest and fair. Over the years they have become almost like family and I've remained with them ever since.

But the ups and downs of this period had some effect on me. I had some swallowing difficulties, for which I had every test under the sun. My senior partner sent me to specialists; I had X-rays but nothing was found.

He called me into his surgery one evening after the latest batch of investigation results came in, all negative again.

'You know what the problem is, my lad?' he said.

'I wish I did,' I replied.

'I think it's this little bit of bother you've had with the magazine. Once you've left all that behind I think your troubles will leave you.'

There was a period of fifteen years from when I started offering my series of anecdotal, humorous medical articles as a possible book, until they actually appeared in book form.

I had literally dozens of rejections, and the trauma of this inexplicable experience with the editors from this leading magazine. Yet, whenever I go to a writing weekend or to a writer's conference, my fellow writers will quite rightly say to me, 'God, you're lucky to get books published.'

There are a few requisites needed to become an established writer and to have books published, but you don't require great gifts, or even great skills.

What has never been told before is *your* story in *your* own words.

What you need is perseverance; of course, luck is an essential; and, if you are really lucky, a good agent.

It was interesting that the national Sunday that serialised my first book said they would be happy to serialise any subsequent book of the same type. However, when the second book appeared, they didn't like it, gave it a terrible review and didn't serialise it. The third book they gave a good review to, but no further serialisations.

Subsequent books have been serialised in other British magazines, and in New

Zealand, Holland, Denmark, and there were German editions of the first four books of the series, plus paperback and large print editions.

I have been very lucky.

13

Full Circle

THERE'S little doubt when I look back over my life that some of the happiest times have been spent on holiday with the children, taking them to new, exciting places.

Children, of course, grow up and from sixteen onwards they tend to go on holiday on their own. Ours were very good and for many years continued the pattern, finding a spare week so that we could have a family get-together in some holiday situation.

Nowadays, holidays are no longer family affairs, and Pam and I tend to go off on our own or with a couple of friends.

The arrival of Daisy May, our first grandchild, provided the opportunity for family holidays again, and we, as doting grandparents, could offer the added service of mobile baby-sitting.

We had done some scouting in France and on a holiday with Jim and Tighe Reeves had found a delightful place in Dinard, Hotel Les Pins, which consisted of about a dozen very well-equipped apartments in a converted farmhouse.

There were all sorts of facilities — an indoor games room with Space Invaders, darts, table tennis and billiards; some lovely grounds and a big barbecue area at the back. There was, of course, a place for playing *boule*, and for a special Breton game in which you threw metal discs on to a board. In the evenings you could come down to a communal lounge which had its own bar.

The thing that made this particular place so attractive were the proprietors, Monsieur and Madame Perrier (as in Perrier water). They were absolutely delightful, nothing was too much trouble. They were always at hand for a chat, help and advice. They even produced a syringe for me to unblock one of Pam's ears. We had a maid service, we could have had petit déjeuner (breakfast) in the small restaurant there. If we wanted, bread would be delivered each day.

Monsieur Perrier's great love was fishing and a day's free fishing was thrown in with every fortnight's stay, or you could organise private trips with him. His boat was his pride and joy.

The farmhouse was on the top of a hill just outside Dinard. Being in the country it was completely quiet, and it was less than half a mile from the nearest beach.

We booked the biggest apartment they had, which was a six-berther, for the second half of May and the first half of June.

One of the many advantages of Dinard is the fact that it's only a few miles from the port of St Malo, and we hoped that family and friends would come to stay with us, travelling over on a night boat. Thus, they wouldn't have to bring a car as we could pick them up from the port.

We loved the Dinard, Dinan, St Malo area; it is a part of Brittany that never seems to get crowded. There are lots of glorious beaches, and in Dinard itself there is the most marvellous promenade walk for several miles, all on the flat, going right round the town. I remember one visit there with some friends, when we walked past the yacht club one spring evening, and the whole cliff face behind the club was covered in fairy lights and classical music was coming out of a series of loudspeakers along the promenade it was quite delightful.

Pam and I travelled on our own from Portsmouth to Cherbourg. We wanted to be the welcoming party at the apartment as Paul and Gill and Daisy May and Gill's parents, Liz and Eddie, were arriving the next day.

A lovely morning dawned and we drove through the countryside, down to Portsmouth. We were blessed with a smooth ferry crossing, then motored about 150 miles to spend our first night in a quayside hotel at Cancale.

From our hotel bedroom window we could see oyster beds stretching out in the sea, and tractors were busy toing and froing, dragging literally tons of oysters off to local hotels, markets, etc.

The next morning we left early for Dinard as we wanted to call at the hypermarket in St Malo which Gill,

179

my daughter-in-law, thinks is one of the seven wonders of the world. (If she had her own way she would spend her whole holiday there.)

It's absolutely vast — you can buy anything from a car to a packet of peppermints. A huge area is devoted to a fantastic array of foods of every kind, and there are restaurants, and shops for clothes, kitchen and garden equipment . . . everything.

The whole place is immaculate and the service is very pleasant. Moreover most things are inexpensive, particularly the wine. The wine that we bought for under a pound a bottle in the St Malo hypermarket would have cost £5 or £6 in a modest French restaurant.

We had a good hour's shopping in the hypermarket, packing the car with wine, cheese, eggs, etc., then set off for the Hotel Les Pins which was about fifteen minutes drive away.

Our apartment consisted of a huge double bedroom with a six-foot bed and an en-suite toilet and bathroom, a general bathroom, two single beds to be made up in the main living/lounge/dining room, and another room with two bunks in it.

We waited anxiously for Paul, Gill, Liz, Eddie and Daisy May to arrive. It's lovely to show people something new. Like old times, we were back on holiday with the children again.

On the first night, the Perriers invited us to have a drink with them and, realising there were three pairs of adults, offered us, for very little extra money, a double bedroom next door to our apartment, so Liz and Eddie could have more room and privacy.

We all had a great time. Liz and Eddie had spent most of their time in India and this was their first visit to France for many years, although Eddie, in his younger days as a jockey, had ridden at Deauville. Paul, who is a bad traveller, had taken the shortest sea crossing, via Dover to Calais, and he and Gill had spent two days en route having a look round before joining us at Dinard. They had spent one night in Honfleur and one in Amboise, an island on which we had camped when Paul was a small boy.

Dinard was full of interesting things: a market twice a week, lovely walks, bays, beaches and shops. One day we took the ferry to the old walled town of St Malo where we lunched, Daisy May enjoying every minute of it. We went down to the golden sands of Sable d'Or, then, after a week, Paul and Gill drove Liz and Eddie back to Cherbourg for their return home, and the next day we picked up Jane from St Malo. She just had three days with us there, but somehow time has no real measurement — it could have been three hours or three weeks.

Although the apartment was well equipped for self-catering we sometimes ate out, most often at the Hotel de Paix in the town. This was an old family hotel which had a very comprehensive menu that worked out at about £5 a head. It had a nice atmosphere and would have cost three times as much for its English equivalent.

Paul and Gill are superb cooks and really went to town with all the exotic food they could buy in the Dinard shops and markets.

We reluctantly said goodbye to Jane and then a few days later we had to wave farewell to Paul and Gill. Before they left we went for a splendid lunch at Erquy, further down the coast, where we sat on the top floor of a restaurant and had a superb meal as we watched the fishing boats come into the harbour. It's a large fishing port and as you look out over the main harbour wall you could see bay after bay along the coastline.

We weren't alone for long. A couple of days later I went down to the St Malo ferry to pick up Margaret and Terry and their son Nigel. Margaret types my books.

They also loved Dinard, especially the Hotel Les Pins, and we went with them to some of the places we discovered with Paul and Gill. Further along the coast we found a marvellous view from Cap Frehel. On one or two occasions we went walking with different visitors and scrambled over Fort le Latte.

Margaret and Terry thought they'd had their best French meal ever in the Hotel de Paix, and they made up their minds to come back to Hotel Les Pins again.

I think there's a lot to be said for a short holiday. By virtue of special travel concessions on the Portsmouth to St Malo ferry, Jane and Margaret's family were able to enjoy France and then return on the night of the third day, which worked out at less than staying in a two-star English hotel for a weekend.

The last couple to join us were our old neighbours, Stan and Pauline Williams, who came for ten days, bringing their Range Rover.

Outings were split between my little Ford and, for the longer journeys, Stan's Range Rover. In the latter, being higher up, we got a much better view of the countryside.

We'd been to Dinard with Stan and Pauline before, so with Stan driving we ventured further afield. One day we travelled eastwards, following the coastline, past St Brieuc as far as Morlaix, exploring as we went. Perhaps the most picturesque stretch was the Baie d'Lannion which ran from St Michel en Grove to St Eclamp. It was a long day's drive, but worth it.

Having more time, we were also able to fulfil one of our ambitions, which was to catch the ferry that plied from St Malo to Dinard, and up the River

Rance to Dinan and back. On reflection I think we should have taken the boat just one way and come back by bus, but we'd booked a return and there was a bar that served drinks and coffee, which was some consolation. The River Rance is cut off from the St Malo/Dinard bay by a great barrage and tidal power station which I believe is the only one of its kind in France.

We boarded the steamer with about a hundred school children and passed through one side of the barrier, then on past a whole number of riverside towns and marinas, right up into the town of Dinan itself. Or rather to the lower part of Dinan where we could get out and have a meal before the boat turned round and went back. The main town of Dinan is on top of a hill. What we hadn't appreciated was that on the way back, the boat went to St Malo before it went to Dinard, which made the journey longer. There was only one small problem; I found the steps from the ferry station at Dinard up to the top road pretty hard going; there were hundreds of them, but I made it all right with a bit of puffing and panting.

On Pentecost Sunday we went to Sable d'Or for a special meal at a hotel. We knew it would be difficult to get in somewhere, so we'd booked ahead all the young confirmants were out having great family meals.

In the hotel there was one little boy who was king for the day, with thirty or forty relatives all dining together after his confirmation. Their meal included a special cake which looked like a mountain of profiteroles. Everybody was dressed in his or her Sunday best, except one or two rather countrified gentlemen, probably farmers, firmly keeping their hats (trilbies or flat caps) on throughout the festivities.

After Stan and Pauline had gone, the next day Pam and I wandered round the town — we had just two or three days left to ourselves. We followed the promenade east out of Dinard, finding new bays and beaches that we'd never discovered before. We had parked our car in the town and had noticed a GB plate on a car parked a few yards from ours. When we returned to our car the other GB people were heading back to theirs, and lo and behold it was my midwife from Tadchester, Amanda Leak (our 'leaky midwife' as I called her), with her husband and very tiny baby.

So we had a day with them and they came back to Hotel Les Pins. They'd brought a caravan across and had all sorts of hair-raising adventures, and finished up based at Dole. They had heard on the grapevine that we were in Dinard.

We had a splendid holiday. I'd bathed in the sea with Jane, we'd got to know our granddaughter, who was a little angel, all our guests had been good fun, and most of them were good cooks, particularly Paul, Liz and Gill.

There was an abundance of *fruits de mer* in Dinard. The fishermen seemed very busy all the time, with boats coming and going, and fish and shellfish pouring in. We had the most gorgeous prawns and mussels, as well as fresh strawberries and always a plentiful supply of wine. Somehow the French seemed to have learnt how to live better and more fully then we do.

Dinard was neat and tidy, and its

harbour absolutely chockablock with boats of every sort. It was nice to drive down to the end of one beach and see the boats come in; sometimes there'd be a passenger liner moored in the bay. We'd watch the Brittany ferry boats coming in and out in the morning and evening, and we'd see the Emerard ferry coming from the Channel Islands, as well as various cargo boats. The place was alive and there was something to see all the time. I would love a little apartment overlooking the bay where I could just sit and watch. Who knows? Some day . . .

Besides dining out at the Hotel de Paix, we also explored one or two other restaurants at various prices. At one, according to our translation, we ordered half a crab mayonnaise. We had a great shock when the dish arrived. There were two huge spider crabs and a whole set of instruments, and we had to get cracking and find the crabmeat ourselves. This involved a lot of hard work with only a little reward!

When we used to go seine-net fishing in Tadchester, we used to put the spider crabs back in the sea; they weren't eaten back there. But everything that moves in France gets eaten. We had a good laugh and I must have had at least a teaspoonful of crabmeat.

Dinard has many beaches and on the main one, where in summer the whole of the promenade is filled with tables and chairs, you can get any sort of meal. There's a huge flat expanse of beach and at low tide land yachts race to and fro. There's an ice-cream parlour tucked away in a sheltered corner, where everybody who is anybody goes with their dogs for morning tea or coffee or an ice-cream, and there are a couple of little cafés which seem to be open all the year round.

We had a splendid time. On our last night at Hotel Les Pins the Perriers asked us to join them in a bottle of champagne. Their daughter was just off to America and we'd already fixed for her friend, Patricia, to come and stay with Paul and Gill for a couple of weeks to learn a bit of English and see something of England. We hoped to see her too, and promised her a trip on the Thames.

One great surprise at the Hotel Les

Pins was when Margaret brought with her a new German edition of one of my books. There were mainly German guests at the hotel and one of them recognised the book.

It had always been my ambition to find somebody who'd read one of my books, or to see someone actually reading one. It was strange that I'd at last found a fan club.

One family of Germans I met in Dinard possessed all the German editions of my books at home and knew all about our family. They would ask Pam questions like, 'Did your father really do this or that?' and 'How is Paul?' and 'What's Trevor doing?' and I know that from now on I shall have a regular sale of at least four German books every time I have one printed over there.

We set off home reluctantly. We had had a really good time and even having been there for a month, would have been happy to stay on. We were looking forward to seeing our dog, Bertie. We knew he was in good hands because 'Our Norman' looked after him and the house while we were away.

We had a good crossing but driving back through England we couldn't help noticing how we English don't seem to bother about the verges or the cleanliness of the roadsides nearly as much as the French do.

I remember being particularly impressed by a group of tall, bronzed men in skimpy bathing trunks who walked up and down the promenade at Dinard with a shovel and brush. At first I thought they were life guards. Then I thought they were collecting litter, but I was wrong — they were there purely for picking up dog dirt and there was a notice that dogs were not allowed on the beach.

I couldn't see that happening in England and I knew that Bertie certainly wouldn't have approved of it.

Anyway, *vive la France* . . . *vive l'entente cordial*. We shall certainly go there again.

14

Cheap at Half the Price

EVERY spring it has been our custom to go on a river trip with our friends Joe and Lyn Church. This year we were having to postpone it as their younger daughter, Catherine, was to be married in June and Lyn would need at least six months time for a nervous breakdown before the wedding occurred. (This is completely untrue — she is one of the calmest, nicest people anyone could meet anywhere.)

We were invited to the wedding; it only made me feel old. Both Catherine and Julie, the Church's two daughters, were my babies. I had looked after Lyn during her pregnancies and had delivered Julie at home in a small cottage on the side of a steep hill in Tadchester. Now here she was, a tall, striking blonde, a very capable business woman, in fact, an absolute stunner.

I'd have to see if I could get her paired off with Trevor.

Catherine wasn't my baby in the fact that I hadn't delivered her as I had Julie. She was born in Winchcombe Hospital, but I did look after Lyn before and after delivery and saw Catherine a few hours after she was born, never realising she would turn into the gorgeous bride I was seeing today.

Catherine was marrying an old college friend, Richard, and they had the great advantage that he and his parents have started from scratch and built up the most superb hotel near Tetbury in Gloucester. In just three years the hotel had earned itself a Michelin star.

In our younger days, Joe, Lyn, Pam and I used to go seine-net fishing in the surf at Sanford-on-Sea. Later, we'd gone boating together, never at any time really snappily dressed. Now, here we all were, gathered on a most beautiful sunny day, in grey toppers and tails. I can't remember going to a nicer wedding in a nicer setting. The church was about eight miles outside Tetbury, a little Norman church surrounded by lovely stone buildings. It was so tiny that they had to put nameplaces where people sat and the curate of the parish, who was to marry them, was in fact, an elderly bishop, complete with his bishop's regalia. He was a bit out of touch with conducting wedding services, he said, having not done one for a year or two, and it was a little confusing when we were asked to pray and sing a hymn at the same time, but in some way it added to the sweetness of the occasion.

The day was absolutely glorious, one of those golden sunny days when everything in England looks green and fresh and nothing in the world can really compare with it. Unfortunately sunshine like this in our country is only too rare.

The bridegroom, Richard, must have been very popular as he had great difficulty in deciding who were going to be his ushers, in the end he had thirteen and they worked like a well-trained set of guardsmen. They were all over the place, they showed us where our car had to be parked, directed us out of the car park after the service, then all the way along the route to the reception there were signs and ushers until we pulled in to a most beautiful Cotswolds stone hotel. Outside, on a huge expanse of lawn, a jazz band that Catherine had spotted in Bristol, were playing to the guests.

As we arrived white-coated waiters welcomed us with glasses of Bucks Fizz.

It was a really special day. If you'd tried to make a film set out of an English wedding in an English country house on a lovely summer's day, you couldn't have bettered this.

The rest of the wedding kept up this standard. The wedding breakfast was out of this world, and included a most beautiful coloured patterned pâté, and salmon specially brought up from the River Tad and cooked in pastry. One of the nicest things was that all the employees, waiters, cooks, chefs at the hotel were all part of the wedding itself.

Lyn looked quite gorgeous in a wide-brimmed hat and summer dress. I'd only seen her in jumpers and jeans before. Joe, a most accomplished lecturer and speaker, usually about birds of prey, proved that he was an even better and funnier speaker at a wedding breakfast giving away his daughter, without ever once mentioning his hobbyhorse, river pollution.

We didn't know many people there but we knew both Joe and Lyn's mothers and we met a whole host of new people, friends who came from Holland, and of course, the thirteen ushers.

The food and wine were excellent and, as it happened, I was sitting next to a man who valued it as highly as I did, and he should have known, as for twelve years he had owned a very up-market West Country hotel.

He told me that he was judged to have the most comprehensive wine list in the West of England with prices ranging from £3 or £4 to £200 a bottle.

I've always been curious about expensive wine and asked him, 'Who would buy a bottle of wine for £150? Was it worth it or just snobbery?'

He doubted if it was even worth spending more than £10 or £15 for a bottle unless you were one of that exceedingly small, well-endowed group who had such cultivated palates that even minor changes in taste and bouquet could be of great meaning. What used to grieve him, he said, were businessmen entertaining other businessmen on expense accounts where £100 bottles of wine would be bought to impress, and at the end of the evening the wines had not been properly appreciated and half-empty bottles littered the table.

He said it was usually the people who made the least fuss about the wine who knew the most about it, and he explained that a good wine for you was the one you liked best. He felt there was a great deal of snob value attached to many wines: many people did not know whether they were enjoying a wine until they'd read the label.

He told me, 'The shorter in supply any particular wine is, the greater the demand for it and the greater the virtues placed upon it.'

It reminded me of corned beef. The British tommy of World War I virtually fought the whole of the war on corned beef and, now, through various market variations, corned beef is really a delicacy. I've always loved it, irrespective of the price; it used to be my favourite school dinner.

My wine-expert companion told me that once a year the managing director of one of England's biggest wine importers would come to stay for a single night in his hotel. This was an annual trip to check on some of his company's warehouses a few miles away. On the first occasion my neighbour watched with interest when this 'king of wine' went in to dinner. He wondered what he would order to drink.

To his great surprise the gentleman chose his cheapest wine, a claret costing £3.70.

This seemed utterly amazing. This particular guest certainly wasn't short of funds; he was a wealthy man in his own right and, anyway, you could rest assured that his trip was being paid for by the firm.

My friend was completely puzzled and made a mental note to try the wine himself. However, other events intervened and he forgot all about it until the following year, when the wine company MD came down for his annual visit.

When the managing director went in to dinner, once again he ordered the cheapest claret.

The hotelier went down to his cellar and found that he had several cases of this wine. He opened a bottle, tasted it and found it was absolutely superb. He couldn't think why he'd never tried it before: in all probability it was because it was the cheapest wine on his list.

He approached the managing director after his meal and said, 'Sir, I do apologise for being so personal, but I've noticed that each time you stay you buy a bottle of our cheapest wine. I've just tried it and it's absolutely superb; as good a wine as I've ever tasted.'

The managing director, with a twinkle in his eye, said, 'You are absolutely right. It's really a trade secret, but my fellow directors and I decided that we would put ourselves in the position of being able to afford to buy the wine we like whenever we stayed out of London at some up-market hotel. So we priced one of our choicest wines at a very low price and made sure it was stocked at the very best hotels.' He added, 'I think that we're the only people who drink it. After all, if you're entertaining an important client and are given a wine list with a price range of £3.70 to £150, it's unlikely that you would go for the bottle priced at £3.70.'

There's a moral in this story somewhere, but the greatest tragedy is that although the hotelier divulged the name of this most precious wine, I failed to write it down and I have forgotten it.

We lingered on after the wedding breakfast, walking round the grounds of this lovely hotel. We saw Catherine and Richard off on their honeymoon, their car was covered with lipstick, balloons, confetti and all the usual paraphernalia that young people try to embarrass each other with at going away times. They were to have a motoring holiday in France, staying at a lot of prime eating and drinking places.

It was a great occasion and we saw them off in a cloud of confetti.

We'd had lots and lots of photographs taken outside the church and in the grounds when we arrived. The poor photographer was still rushing around

— he hadn't taken a photograph of the ushers.

Eventually after much hard work by Joe and Catherine's father-in-law, all thirteen ushers were rounded up.

The photographer, anxious to be off, said, 'Come now, gentlemen, adopt a relaxed pose.'

Immediately, all the ushers, for some reason, loosened their waistbands, and kept moving about until eventually he got them settled.

'Right, gentlemen,' he said, 'smile for the camera. Ready, steady, go,' and at the word 'go' he clicked his camera, to be beaten by all the ushers dropping their trousers and showing thirteen pairs of Union Jack underpants.

The place was in an uproar, but somehow it was the perfect end to a perfect British wedding in the perfect British house on a perfect British day.

15

Changing Direction

I'D been feeling off-colour for a while, not really ill, but was having all sorts of odd aches and pains in my chest. There must have been reasons for them but I tended to dismiss them.

We had a late boat holiday in October with our friends Lyn and Joe Church. Their daughter's wedding in the spring had prevented our usual trip and although Pam and I have had excellent boating holidays in October, this particular one with Joe and Lyn struck a patch of mid-winter. It was cold, wet and rainy with a very strong wind. We passed down river, missing the best of that most glorious stretch of river, the Goring Gap, where tree-lined slopes come down to the river's edge, because we were stuck inside as wind and rain buffeted the boat. The weather cleared a bit towards the evening and we found a mooring some way below

Whitchurch Lock.

It was warm in the boat but it was so wet everywhere we were wandering around in oilskins. The weather forecast promised some improvement.

We cast off the next morning under gloomy skies and went through Mapledurham Lock. The last time we'd been through here it had been flooded and the whole lock was under water. We motored on through a grey-looking Reading, one of the few industrial areas of the Thames. At Caversham Lock we renewed our acquaintance with the lock keeper, with whom we'd travelled in convoy up the river the year before, when he was taking his boat up for a month on the canals. Then down on to picturesque Sonning Lock looking for the spot where we'd been stuck for three days when the river had been flooded. We remembered that we'd rung home to tell them we were all right, only to be told that Trevor had fallen in Sark and had broken his thigh.

We continued on in poor weather and moored early, not out in the country as is our usual wont, but at the upper end of the park in Henley. I was a bit cold so stayed in the boat while the others went off to explore the town. There was still plenty of room for the dogs, Bertie and Jenny, to run around but it wasn't the sort of country they really like.

It was raining when we set off the following morning, passing under Henley Bridge and through the lovely broad sweep of river there. We moved on to Hambledon Lock, then to Temple Lock, where we called in on our friends, Bob Munro Ashman and his wife Sian. I'd borrowed two of Bob's books by Fred Archer, the old authority on the Thames, and I'd promised to take them down by boat. Bob had been a neighbour of ours in Wallingford when he was relief lock keeper on Cleeve, Goring and Benson Locks. Temple Lock was the first lock of his own and he seemed very happy there. Meanwhile it was still pouring with rain. Bob was optimistic; there was a good chance of it clearing up.

We continued on down river, through Marlow, passing, as we approached Marlow Lock, the huge weir stream that ran for several hundred yards on one side of the river. We somehow chugged through Cookham without even noticing, because before we knew where we were, we were in Cookham Lock. The stretch from Marlow to Cookham is unattractive compared with the Thames up river. The river's so wide you feel you're at sea and there's a lot of river development. Although there are some pretty parts, it's all rather drab.

Leaving Cookham Lock we entered what I consider is the most beautiful stretch of the river and this was our main objective, Cliveden Reach. We'd originally intended to spend a night there but it was blowing a gale so we moored up on one of the many islands, had lunch and cruised down as far as Boulters Lock and started on our return journey. It was quite lovely, with wooded slopes going up to Cliveden and clusters of islands. All through this stretch you could moor and have your own island. The dogs adored it.

Just after leaving Cookham Lock, the boat suddenly lost power; we hardly made any headway at all. There was a huge crosswind and it was pouring with rain — we were at a loss as to what to do. We debated whether to go into a boat yard, wondering if the clutch was slipping.

The stretch from Cookham Lock to Marlow took us over two hours. When I looked at the bank sometimes we didn't appear to be moving at all. We decided to negotiate Marlow Lock and then find a boat yard. I'd once had a similar experience when the throttle was slipping but it didn't feel quite like that. I was worried about passing the huge weir stream on our port side just beyond Marlow Lock. With so little headway on we could be in trouble. It seemed hours coming, I was quite dry-mouthed. There were hardly any other boats on the river, and there was a wind sweeping right across it. There was nothing to protect us. The engine could barely keep our nose into the wind.

Eventually, around a bend in the river, there was the shelter of Marlow Lock, and it was open. We pulled in to a perfect stop, with me putting the propeller astern to bring us to a complete halt.

I dreaded what it was going to be like

coming out of the lock.

The lock filled up, the gates opened. I started up the engine and we cruised out, to our amazement, under full power.

'It must have been the clutch not properly engaged,' said Joe.

We pulled clear of the lock and moored up behind a boat with an experienced boatman aboard. He diagnosed our problem: 'You must have had a plastic bag round your propeller and by going astern in the lock you cleared it. You were very lucky.'

Sea Grey was built in such a way that it was extremely difficult to get at the propeller — it would have meant diving down beneath the boat and this wasn't the weather for it. The gale was blowing into the bank here but even so we lashed ourselves to the quayside with about three extra ropes. Joe went into the town to buy a Chinese takeaway and this, washed down with a bottle of wine, seemed to reduce our troubles miraculously.

It was a bit finer the next morning. We set off, with the engine under full power and we made good progress upstream, passing once more through Henley, which is such a lovely sight from the river, up through Shiplake and moored again, as we had on an earlier night, beside the field just below Whitchurch Lock. By now there was a tremendous gale blowing and we hardly dared get out of the boat. (Thank goodness for our inside toilet.)

Joe, mustering every item of waterproof clothing, volunteered to exercise the dogs from time to time. I was complaining to Pam that my chest was uncomfortable. This wasn't really surprising because all the wind and the rain had involved a lot more heaving and pulling than usual, and having had a coronary by-pass operation, the scar often gave discomfort when I did extra or, in particular, different physical movements.

We set off for home early next morning, passing Whitchurch, Goring, and Cleeve Locks, arriving at our homeward stretch to moor. We unpacked the boat in the pouring rain and I did find it very wearying plodding up and down to the boat with our stores and equipment. We all had a hot bath to revive us, Pam had nipped out for fish and chips, and we all had a good cup of tea, mission accomplished.

'Well,' said Joe, beaming, 'home at last. Do you know what the best part of that trip was?'

'No,' I said.

'The hot bath I've just had.'

I certainly did ache all over through carrying and pulling. It was very difficult holding the boat into the moorings waiting to go through locks. In all it was a very strenuous holiday and I made up my mind that my days of fighting the elements were over.

After the trip I allowed myself a few lazy days. The weather didn't improve much and the following week brought a hurricane.

The day after the hurricane we went down to Brighton to see Trevor and Jane, who had damage to their skylight and Trevor's bedroom window had been knocked out.

Water was pouring in through the skylight. I had brought with me some sheets of rubber and various things I thought might help.

Driving down to Brighton reminded

me of the Blitz. There were trees down everywhere, some lying across houses or cars. The roads were being cleared, but there were literally thousands of trees down; it would be hundreds of years before they could be replaced.

Trevor and I clambered out on to his roof and managed to seal the skylight. It was not an easy task — we were four storeys up and, about four feet away, there was a sharp drop to the ground; it also had such a high sloping roof that we had to hang on to the skylight frame with one hand holding the nails in our teeth.

'Should you be doing that?' said Trevor.

'Yes,' I said, 'I'm as fit as a flea!'

Between us we managed to get things watertight and Trevor fixed the double glazing across his broken window.

We came back home the next day and I had a go at some of my own damaged trees. A few of the willows looked very dangerous and, in spite of Pam's protests, just to show how young and fit I was, I climbed up some of the willows and sawed off great big branches, hanging on upside down with one arm, legs wrapped around the trunk, and sawing in a most difficult position. It was really hard work and at the end of it I'd used more muscles than I had in years and had a corresponding few more aches and pains.

The final straw came when a few days later a man arrived with some books. When a hardback book has gone into paperback and has been published for some time, if all the hardbacks have not been sold, the author has the option of buying them at a very cheap rate. There were four hundred of one of my hardbacks left and I decided to buy the lot.

The delivery man brought seven boxes of books to the door. They must have weighed three-quarters of a hundredweight each; Pam couldn't even lift one off the floor. I not only carried each one upstairs but also climbed the step ladder into the loft, or, shall I say, fought my way up into the loft. Then, once inside the loft, on my hands and knees, I had to lift them over the cross-beams to store them.

I had seven journeys to make and it

really took the stuffing out of me. Again I used muscles I hadn't used for years; my shoulders ached like anything. 'I must be fit if I can do something like this,' I remarked to Pam.

She said, 'I don't know if you're fit or stupid.'

The aches in my chest continued; they weren't specific, nothing like heart trouble. I did go and have a medical check-up and nothing obvious showed up.

One Sunday night I awoke with a pain in my chest that I couldn't ignore and I realised I was having a coronary. The doctor was called and I was whipped off to the Royal Berks Hospital, and it was almost an advantage to have a coronary to experience the monitoring unit they have there. On arrival, a cheerful nurse said, 'Do we address you as Doctor Robert Clifford, Robert or Bob?'

I said, 'Bob.'

She said, 'Right, my name's Gill, this is Ian,' and so on, and in the next few days there I experienced nursing of the highest standard.

The ward was immaculate; everybody

was cheerful; nothing was too much trouble. My symptoms settled down after a couple of days and I was spoilt by being able to stay on in the ward for a bit longer, as for once they weren't pressed for beds.

I have never been so impressed by such a degree of efficiency and care. When you find units of such a high standard there's usually one or two people who are the main motivators behind them. In this case I think there was a doctor and a ward sister who, with their enthusiasm, kept up these exemplary levels of nursing, care, and most important of all, kindness and consideration.

It was a mixed ward. It was very funny being next to a lady — fine when you were chatting, but not quite so fine when you had to have a bedpan with only a curtain to separate you.

On my fourth day I saw a man in the bed opposite me come in and die.

The house surgeon was taking a history from him. The man had been admitted in a lot of pain having had a coronary. He'd been given treatment for his pain, which had settled, but suddenly I saw him go limp and sag over, gone. The houseman kept on talking, then realised his patient was no longer responding. He shouted an order. In a few seconds there was a sound of running feet, of machines, doctors and nurses appearing from all over. I couldn't see what was going on as they drew the curtains, but there was a lot of activity: 'Turn him this way. Give him this. Right, give him one more shot.' They managed to revive him and pull him through this attack, and he was hanging on.

I was moved from the ward the next day but kept an interest in him and saw him improve generally. He was sitting up in bed reading the paper before I left. I was put in the main ward for a couple of days where, again, the nursing was excellent. The sister, who I think was West Indian, said to me, 'There's your bed, Doctor Clifford.'

'Actually, my name's Bob,' I said.

'Not in this ward,' she said. 'I'm one of the old school.' She laughed but she had her ward staff on their toes. Everything was efficient and well run and the nursing auxiliaries and the ladies who brought the tea round added a tremendous amount of colour to the ward. This was not just because they came from India, Pakistan, the West Indies and other far-flung places, but they were lively, smiling people who cheered us up. One nursing auxiliary, a Jamaican, was practically a music-hall turn on her own. We looked forward to her coming in. As well as being entertaining she was a most devoted and caring nurse and couldn't have been kinder or more gentle.

The hospital were very organised about my departure: an outpatients appointment was made, I was given tablets, and it was arranged that the district nurse would call on me. They even let me home a bit early as my new young GP had offered to keep an eye on me at home. I was lucky, I'd had an uncomplicated incident and there was no reason why I shouldn't, after a period of rest, get over it completely and resume most of the things I was doing before.

It was lovely to get home again, lie in my bed and look out at the river flowing past. I got myself an exercise bicycle, and pedalled away each day. It was not long before I was walking into the town, and doing circular trips around the boat yard. I'd been very lucky. I had to take various sorts of medication and it was a little while before we found the one that suited me the best and I fortunately had no further troubles.

My old friend John Bowler came up from Tadchester with his daughter, to stay. *Sea Grey* was out of the water for the winter, looking absolutely huge on the hard-standing in the front garden. I asked him whether my boating days were over.

'Well, I think the time has come to be sensible,' he said. 'Both the episodes you've had, the one before your coronary by-pass and this latest one, have followed periods when you've done some excessive, strenuous physical activity. The first time it was carrying a dinghy on your back and this last time, I think it was carrying those books upstairs. I think you'll be fine providing you don't put yourself under extreme physical pressure. Walking, riding, running, going around, say, in a day boat would be fine. You've got your writing, and there's so much of France you haven't explored yet, but I think you'll really have to give up battling against the elements. Your boat weighs several tons, and if it gets stuck in the mud you'll have to push it off — it's just not worth it. My advice to you is to get rid of it. I know it's a bit sad, but you have so enjoyed your days on the river, it would be a pity to let it damage your health.'

He was right. I knew when we were down on Cliveden Reach that I didn't really want much more of gales, storms and hanging on to moorings for dear life; but it was sad — we'd been so happy and had had such good holidays on the Thames. But there were other things we could do. I have always claimed I had two main loves, the Thames and France; now I would have to concentrate on the latter.

The Williams, our ex-neighbours, had invited us to join them in the spring on a touring holiday in France with me navigating and Stan driving his Range Rover ('the tank' as he called it). I'd just have to accept that I was getting

217

a teeny bit older and mustn't look for physical battles.

The weather picked up in February for a short spell, one of those false springs and it was sunny. There were one or two people out on the river. Pam and I walked down the garden and there was our boat, *Sea Grey*, perched on oil-drums on our hard-standing, covered in the new blue tarpaulin I'd bought at the beginning of the winter to protect her from the worst of the weather.

I tacked a 'For Sale' notice on her; I'd already let the Maid Boat Yard and Andrew Corless at the Sheridan Boat Yard know she was up for sale.

I stood back with Pam, looking at her.

It was sad to think that we'd had our last voyage on her.

Pam squeezed my hand.

'D'you know what?' she said.

'Yes,' I replied, 'You don't have to tell me: life is going to be different from now on.'

Postscript

THERE is the fable of the old man sitting outside a town, being approached by a stranger.

'What are they like in this town?' asked the stranger.

'What were they like in your last town?' replied the old man.

'They were delightful people. I was very happy there. They were kind, generous and would always help you in trouble.'

'You will find them very much like that in this town.'

The old man was approached by another stranger.

'What are the people like in this town?' asked the second stranger.

'What were they like in your last town?' replied the old man.

'It was an awful place. They were mean, unkind and nobody would ever help anybody.'

'I am afraid you will find it very much

219

the same here,' said the old man.

If it should be your lot to ever visit Wallingford, this is how you will find it.

TO FIGHT THE WILD
Rod Ansell and Rachel Percy

Lost in uncharted Australian bush, Rod Ansell survived by hunting and trapping wild animals, improvising shelter and using all the bushman's skills he knew.

COROMANDEL
Pat Barr

India in the 1830s is a hot, uncomfortable place, where the East India Company still rules. Amelia and her new husband find themselves caught up in the animosities which seethe between the old order and the new.

THE SMALL PARTY
Lillian Beckwith

A frightening journey to safety begins for Ruth and her small party as their island is caught up in the dangers of armed insurrection.

FATAL RING OF LIGHT
Helen Eastwood

Katy's brother was supposed to have died in 1897 but a scrawled note in his handwriting showed July 1899. What had happened to him in those two years? Katy was determined to help him.

NIGHT ACTION
Alan Evans

Captain David Brent sails at dead of night to the German occupied Normandy town of St. Jean on a mission which will stretch loyalty and ingenuity to its limits, and beyond.

A MURDER TOO MANY
Elizabeth Ferrars

Many, including the murdered man's widow, believed the wrong man had been convicted. The further murder of a key witness in the earlier case convinced Basnett that the seemingly unrelated deaths were linked.

THE WILDERNESS WALK
Sheila Bishop

Stifling unpleasant memories of a misbegotten romance in Cleave with Lord Francis Aubrey, Lavinia goes on holiday there with her sister. The two women are thrust into a romantic intrigue involving none other than Lord Francis.

THE RELUCTANT GUEST
Rosalind Brett

Ann Calvert went to spend a month on a South African farm with Theo Borland and his sister. They both proved to be different from her first idea of them, and there was Storr Peterson — the most disturbing man she had ever met.

ONE ENCHANTED SUMMER
Anne Tedlock Brooks

A tale of mystery and romance and a girl who found both during one enchanted summer.

CLOUD OVER MALVERTON
Nancy Buckingham

Dulcie soon realises that something is seriously wrong at Malverton, and when violence strikes she is horrified to find herself under suspicion of murder.

AFTER THOUGHTS
Max Bygraves

The Cockney entertainer tells stories of his East End childhood, of his RAF days, and his post-war showbusiness successes and friendships with fellow comedians.

MOONLIGHT AND MARCH ROSES
D. Y. Cameron

Lynn's search to trace a missing girl takes her to Spain, where she meets Clive Hendon. While untangling the situation, she untangles her emotions and decides on her own future.

NURSE ALICE IN LOVE
Theresa Charles

Accepting the post of nurse to little Fernie Sherrod, Alice Everton could not guess at the romance, suspense and danger which lay ahead at the Sherrod's isolated estate.

POIROT INVESTIGATES
Agatha Christie

Two things bind these eleven stories together — the brilliance and uncanny skill of the diminutive Belgian detective, and the stupidity of his Watson-like partner, Captain Hastings.

LET LOOSE THE TIGERS
Josephine Cox

Queenie promised to find the long-lost son of the frail, elderly murderess, Hannah Jason. But her enquiries threatened to unlock the cage where crucial secrets had long been held captive.

THE TWILIGHT MAN
Frank Gruber

Jim Rand lives alone in the California desert awaiting death. Into his hermit existence comes a teenage girl who blows both his past and his brief future wide open.

DOG IN THE DARK
Gerald Hammond

Jim Cunningham breeds and trains gun dogs, and his antagonism towards the devotees of show spaniels earns him many enemies. So when one of them is found murdered, the police are on his doorstep within hours.

THE RED KNIGHT
Geoffrey Moxon

When he finds himself a pawn on the chessboard of international espionage with his family in constant danger, Guy Trent becomes embroiled in moves and countermoves which may mean life or death for Western scientists.

TIGER TIGER
Frank Ryan

A young man involved in drugs is found murdered. This is the first event which will draw Detective Inspector Sandy Woodings into a whirlpool of murder and deceit.

CAROLINE MINUSCULE
Andrew Taylor

Caroline Minuscule, a medieval script, is the first clue to the whereabouts of a cache of diamonds. The search becomes a deadly kind of fairy story in which several murders have an other-worldly quality.

LONG CHAIN OF DEATH
Sarah Wolf

During the Second World War four American teenagers from the same town join the Army together. Forty-two years later, the son of one of the soldiers realises that someone is systematically wiping out the families of the four men.

THE LISTERDALE MYSTERY
Agatha Christie

Twelve short stories ranging from the light-hearted to the macabre, diverse mysteries ingeniously and plausibly contrived and convincingly unravelled.

TO BE LOVED
Lynne Collins

Andrew married the woman he had always loved despite the knowledge that Sarah married him for reasons of her own. So much heartache could have been avoided if only he had known how vital it was to be loved.

ACCUSED NURSE
Jane Converse

Paula found herself accused of a crime which could cost her her job, her nurse's reputation, and even the man she loved, unless the truth came to light.

BUTTERFLY MONTANE
Dorothy Cork

Parma had come to New Guinea to marry Alec Rivers, but she found him completely disinterested and that overbearing Pierce Adams getting entirely the wrong idea about her.

HONOURABLE FRIENDS
Janet Daley

Priscilla Burford is happily married when she meets Junior Environment Minister Alistair Thurston. Inevitably, sexual obsession and political necessity collide.

WANDERING MINSTRELS
Mary Delorme

Stella Wade's career as a concert pianist might have been ruined by the rudeness of a famous conductor, so it seemed to her agent and benefactor. Even Sir Nicholas fails to see the possibilities when John Tallis falls deeply in love with Stella.

CHATEAU OF FLOWERS
Margaret Rome

Alain, Comte de Treville needed a wife to look after him, and Fleur went into marriage on a business basis only, hoping that eventually he would come to trust and care for her.

CRISS-CROSS
Alan Scholefield

As her ex-husband had succeeded in kidnapping their young daughter once, Jane was determined to take her safely back to England. But all too soon Jane is caught up in a new web of intrigue.

DEAD BY MORNING
Dorothy Simpson

Leo Martindale's body was discovered outside the gates of his ancestral home. Is it, as Inspector Thanet begins to suspect, murder?